ELLISON'S
Atlas of surgery
of the
stomach and
duodenum

ELLISON'S
Atlas of surgery of the stomach and duodenum

Larry C. Carey, M.D.

Associate Professor of Surgery
University of Pittsburgh School of Medicine
Pittsburgh, Pennsylvania

Robert H. Albertin, M. A.

Associate Professor and Chairman
Department of Audio-Graphic Communications
The Medical College of Wisconsin
Milwaukee, Wisconsin

With 349 illustrations in 70 plates and 2 figures

The C. V. Mosby Company

Saint Louis   1971

Printed in the United States of America
Standard Book Number 8016-0941-0
Library of Congress Catalog Card Number 76-176386
Distributed in Great Britain by Henry Kimpton, London

CONTRIBUTORS

JOSEPH C. DARIN, M.D.

Professor of Surgery
The Medical College of Wisconsin
Milwaukee, Wisconsin

WILLIAM E. EVANS, M.D.

Associate Professor of Surgery
Ohio State University Medical School
  University Hospital
Columbus, Ohio

RICHARD H. LILLIE, M.D.

Associate Clinical Professor of Surgery
The Medical College of Wisconsin
Milwaukee, Wisconsin

WILLIAM J. SCHULTE, M.D.

Associate Professor of Surgery
The Medical College of Wisconsin
Milwaukee, Wisconsin

THOMAS WALL, M.D.

Assistant Clinical Professor of Surgery
The Medical College of Wisconsin
Milwaukee, Wisconsin

STUART D. WILSON, M.D.

Associate Professor of Surgery
The Medical College of Wisconsin
Milwaukee, Wisconsin

This atlas is dedicated to

Dr. Robert M. Zollinger

because we believe Dr. Ellison would have wished it.

PREFACE

This atlas was the last work of Dr. Edwin H. Ellison. It was begun several years before his death, and it was his intention to provide a detailed description of surgical techniques in treating diseases of the upper abdomen. Dr. Ellison's well-known interest in gastroduodenal and pancreatic disease prompted his desire to contribute an atlas that would be helpful to other surgeons who face problems in these areas. While at Ohio State University he became interested in surgery of hematologic disorders, and the contributions on splenectomy, liver biopsy, and lymph node biopsy stem from that interest.

Dr. Ellison and Mr. Robert Albertin completed most of the illustrative work prior to Dr. Ellison's untimely death. The text of this volume was contributed by men whom Dr. Ellison trained, with the exception of Dr. Richard Lillie, who was his respected colleague and friend.

It was Dr. Ellison's conviction that technical surgery was an art form to be accomplished by skilled professionals. This belief in no way detracted from his emphasis on sound clinical judgment and a compassionate bedside manner. Above all he believed that surgery should be safe. The numerous illustrations were chosen to make certain that the most minute steps of each procedure were shown.

It is the ardent hope of the contributors that we have done justice to "the Boss." We further hope that his wish to contribute a useful volume to assist surgeons in improving the care of their patients has been fulfilled.

Larry C. Carey

CONTENTS

PLATES

ELLISON'S
Atlas of surgery
of the
stomach and
duodenum

CHAPTER
1

Surgical approach to the stomach and related viscera

The position of the patient on the operating table is of critical importance. Maximum comfort for the patient will avoid postoperative backache and muscle soreness. It is the surgeon's responsibility to avoid complications of position such as nerve palsies and pressure necrosis. The efficiency of the surgeon is enhanced if he is able to be comfortable during the procedure. House officers must recognize that attention to these seemingly unimportant details is the first step in developing the attitude that the craft of surgery demands.

PLATE 1 • POSITION OF THE PATIENT AND CHOICE OF INCISION

A Note that the patient has been moved toward the foot of the table so that the kidney rest *(1)* is under the xiphoid process. This greatly facilitates the exposure of upper abdominal organs. This position is used for most upper abdominal procedures and has its greatest application in dealing with those organs that rest near the posterior abdominal wall, such as the adrenals. It is frequently necessary to insert a foot extension at the bottom end of the table to achieve this position. It is also important that the patient be placed as near the right edge of the operating table as possible so that the distance reached by the operating surgeon is reduced to a minimum. To avoid pressure on the ulnar nerve from the kidney rest, the patient's right arm is taped across his body *(2)*. This is accomplished with a piece of 3-inch adhesive tape placed from just above the elbow obliquely across the opposite thigh and fixed to the patient's thigh or to the edge of the operating table, whichever is more convenient. This avoids the necessity of having the patient's arm out to the side and also avoids the problem of pressure from the kidney rest. This has been an extremely useful maneuver and greatly lessens the discomfort of the second assistant. Note that the table is in slight Trendelenburg position, which allows the intra-abdominal organs to fall into the pelvis, exposing more easily the organs in the upper abdomen.

B In this illustration the kidney rest is not being employed. Again note the slight Trendelenburg position of the table and that the patient's right arm has been fixed with adhesive tape to his thigh *(1)*. In this instance an added precaution has been taken by placing a cloth pad posterior to the elbow *(2)*. The positioning of the arm in this manner has virtually eliminated the bracheal plexus injuries associated with the arm being abducted.

C Nearly all surgery of the upper abdomen can be accomplished through a midline incision. This incision is preferred to the pararectus because it is more quickly made and more quickly closed. In general, the peritoneum is closed with interrupted 4-0 silk sutures and the midline fascia with interrupted 2-0 silk sutures. In patients in whom dehiscence is a substantial risk, interrupted wire may be used instead of 2-0 silk on the fascia. Note that the incision has been extended up to the left of the xiphoid, an important maneuver providing a significant increase in exposure for upper abdominal exploration.

D An alternative for the midline incision is the bilateral subcostal incision, which is of particular advantage in patients with widely flaired costal margins.

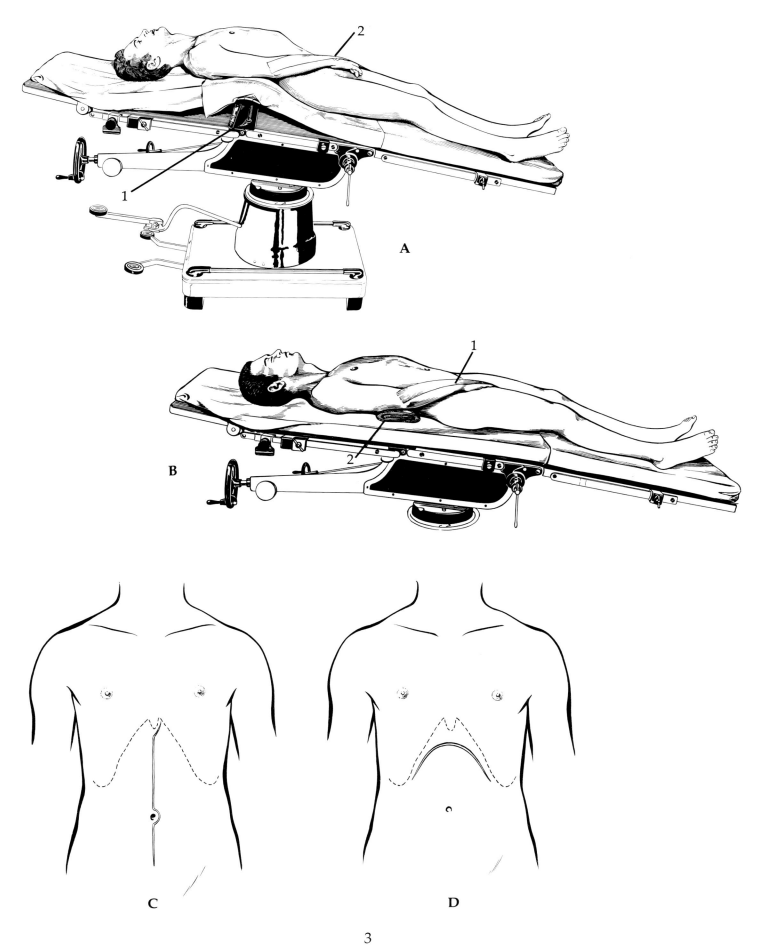

A

B

C

D

2

Mobilization of the stomach, vagotomy, subtotal gastrectomy, and gastroduodenostomy

Hemigastrectomy and vagotomy is the treatment of choice for peptic ulceration of the duodenum as well as peptic ulceration of the stomach in those patients who are hypersecretors of hydrochloric acid.

PLATE 2 • SUBDIAPHRAGMATIC VAGOTOMY

The abdomen has been thoroughly explored. Visual and manual inspection of the area of suspected ulceration has been accomplished, and the decision has been made to proceed with vagotomy and hemigastrectomy. The key to successful and uncomplicated gastric resection lies in adequate mobilization of the stomach.

A The procedure begins with exposure of the gastroesophageal area in preparation for vagotomy. With laparotomy pads *(1)* on the abdominal incision and with the incision held open by self-retaining retractor, a Richardson retractor *(2)* is placed beneath the left subcostal margin, and gentle traction is used to expose the left lobe of the liver. After the left lobe of the liver has been grasped in the right hand, with the thumb anterior to the left lobe and the fingers posterior, the triangular ligament *(3)* is easily exposed. It can usually be seen to be a thin membranous structure containing no blood vessels. With gentle inferior traction on the left lobe of the liver, the triangular ligament is stretched tautly, and with the long dissecting scissors in the left hand of the surgeon, an incision is made in the midportion of the triangular ligament and extended laterally to the edge of the left lobe. After this portion of the left lobe has been mobilized, the retracting hand and the dissecting hand are reversed.

B The left hand is now pulling the left lobe of the liver inferiorly, again putting tension on the triangular ligament. With the dissecting scissors in the right hand, the triangular ligament is further divided medially toward the vena cava. As one approaches the cava, the triangular ligament will be noted to split into an anterior and a posterior leaf, leaving a bare area on the liver. It is about 1 cm. past this point at which this division of the ligament stops. Care must be exercised to avoid injuring the phrenic vessels that are in close proximity to the area of dissection. Should these vessels be injured, the bleeding can generally be controlled easily with a suture ligature. After mobilization of the left lobe has been accomplished, the left lobe is folded gently toward the right, covered with a laparotomy pad, and held with a Deaver retractor.

C A Babcock clamp *(1)* is then placed on the midanterior portion of the stomach, and gentle traction inferiorly assists in exposure of the gastroesophageal junction *(2)*. The peritoneum overlying the gastroesophageal junction is grasped by the forceps, and dissection is begun with the dissecting scissors.

D After the peritoneum has been divided over the gastroesophageal junction, the dissection is continued to the left, dividing the splenorenal ligament *(1)*. This is an important consideration because subsequent traction on the stomach has the potential hazard of tearing the capsule of the spleen *(2)*. If this mobilization procedure has been executed properly, this danger is avoided.

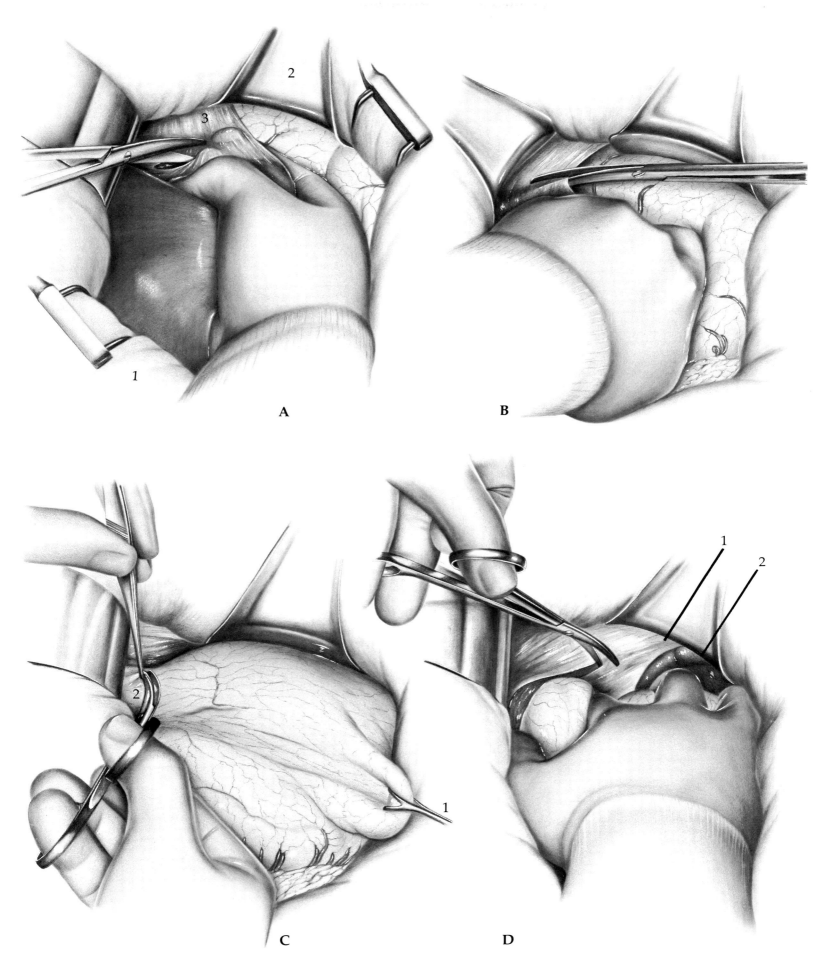

A

B

C

D

7

PLATE 3 • SUBDIAPHRAGMATIC VAGOTOMY—cont'd

A After the peritoneum has been divided over the esophagus, blunt dissection with the index finger is begun to the left of the esophagus. As the finger is introduced into the areolar tissue around the esophagogastric junction, the esophagus is freed from its surrounding loose attachments as it comes through the hiatus of the diaphragm *(1)*. Again the exposure is excellent, with the left lobe of the liver retracted medially *(2)*, and with the left subcostal margin retracted superiorly. Gentle constant traction is maintained inferiorly on the stomach, and the majority of this traction is accomplished with the middle finger of the surgeon's right hand. By continuing the traction on the stomach as the esophagus is freed from the surrounding tissue, the anterior vagus often becomes readily identifiable.

B A right-angle clamp has been placed underneath the anterior vagus trunk *(1)*, and the trunk has been elevated from the esophageal wall. Care must be exercised in the employment of the right-angle clamp, since the sharp tip may easily penetrate the esophageal wall. However, a minimum amount of caution avoids this potential complication.

C Once the anterior trunk has been separated from the esophageal wall, it is divided with the scissors. It is not usually necessary to ligate the vagal trunk unless there is doubt as to whether or not this structure is indeed a vagus nerve. Experience with this dissection leads one to quickly recognize the vagus from other possible anatomic structures, such as a branch of the left gastric artery, and the need for ligation is rare. An additional safety feature is the division of the vagal trunk well toward the gastric aspect of the dissection so that if there is an arterial vessel in the tissue which is divided, it does not retract into the posterior mediastinum, making its subsequent retrieval difficult.

D The index finger *(1)* of the surgeon's right hand is seen posterior to the gastric wall. The index finger and thumb are used to roll the esophagus so that the posterior aspect of the organ *(2)* becomes readily visible in the operative field. Again a right-angle clamp introduced beneath the palpable posterior vagal trunk demonstrates the vagal trunk nicely *(3)*. It is in this area of dissection that truncal vagotomy is often incomplete. With constant traction of the stomach inferiorly, the index finger and thumb are used to explore thoroughly the posterior esophageal tissues. If a vagal trunk is present, it will be felt as a tight band extending from the posterior mediastinum down onto the gastric wall. The key to locating the vagal trunks, and they are often multiple, is the downward traction on the stomach, which tightens the vagal trunks and makes them easily palpable. Blood vessels and strands of muscle from the esophageal hiatus do not develop the tautness that is characteristic of the vagal trunk. After the two major vagal trunks *(3, 4)* have been divided, the esophagus is rolled back and forth between the thumb and index finger, again maintaining constant traction on the stomach downward. Frequently the surgeon will find multiple small strands of vagal tissue that are identified by their tendency to indent the esophageal wall. These are also dissected free from the esophagus with the right-angle clamp and are divided.

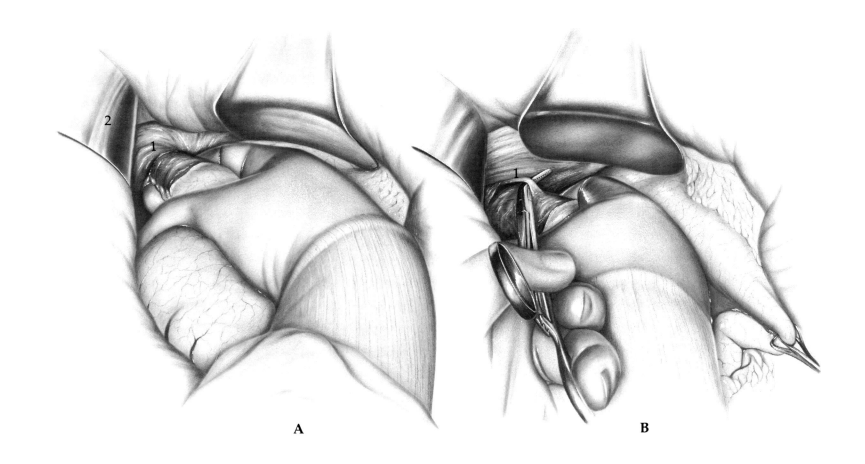

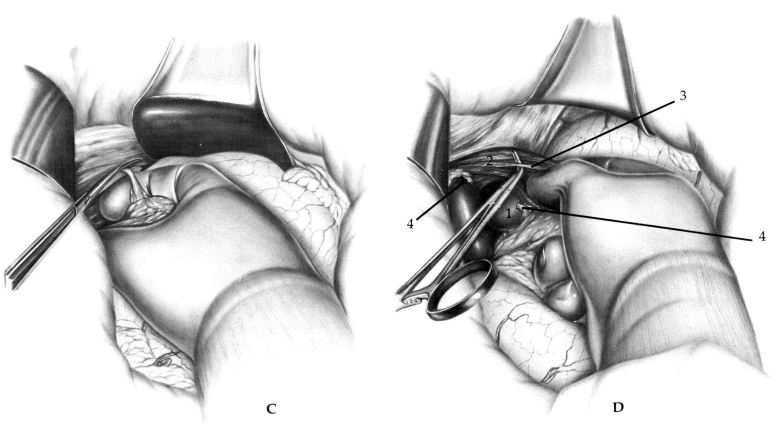

A

B

C

D

9

PLATE 4 • SUBDIAPHRAGMATIC VAGOTOMY—cont'd

A The division of an additional accessory vagus trunk *(1)* is demonstrated here.

B Once the surgeon has been assured of the completeness of the vagotomy, a narrow Deaver retractor *(1)* is placed posterior to the esophagus on the right side, and the organ is retracted superiorly and to the left, exposing the esophageal hiatus *(2)*. Customarily the edges of the esophageal hiatus are reapproximated posteriorly to the esophagus, restoring a hiatal opening that just admits the esophagus. Although this step may not be essential, it is easily accomplished and restores the anatomic arrangement previous to its disruption. Note the segment of esophagus *(3)* that is now residing within the abdominal cavity after truncal vagotomy. It is important to note that 2 to 3 inches of esophagus have been withdrawn from the posterior mediastinum into the abdominal cavity, considerably lengthening the intra-abdominal esophagus and further aiding in the mobilization of the stomach for the subsequent gastroduodenal anastomosis. This maneuver also lessens the risk of esophageal reflux.

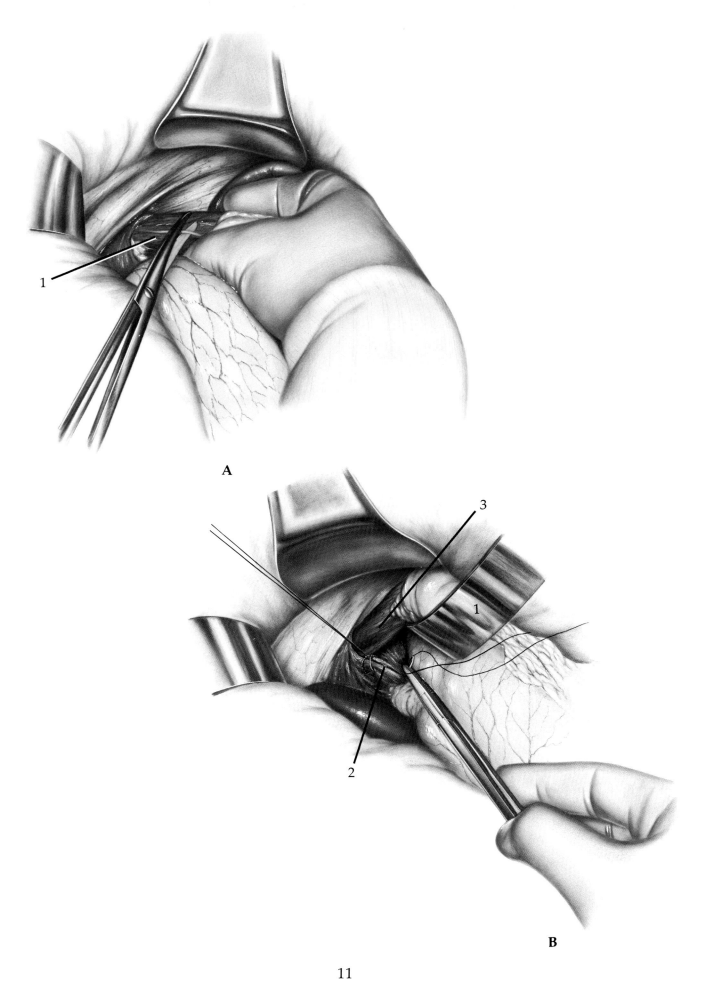

A

B

11

PLATE 5 • SUBTOTAL GASTRECTOMY

This plate demonstrates a variety of methods of handling the vagal trunks in truncal vagotomy.

A The surgeon's right hand has been used to grasp the stomach, with the fingers posterior to the esophagus and the thumb on the anterior aspect of the gastro-esophageal junction. Again the anterior vagal trunk (1) can be seen overlying the esophagus after the peritoneum has been divided.

B The elevation of this anterior vagus with a right-angle clamp and division with with the dissecting scissors can be seen as previously described. Again notice that the vagal division is carried out well below the entrance of the vagus into the abdominal cavity to prevent the retraction into the posterior mediastinum.

C An alternative method is to place hemostatic neurosurgical clips (1) on the vagal trunks prior to division to avoid any potential hemorrhage. This is not done routinely.

D Cross-clamping of the anterior vagal trunk between hemostatic clamps prior to division with the scissors is shown. This procedure allows removal of a segment of the vagus nerve for histologic section, if the surgeon feels insecure about the identity of the trunk, and also allows for ligature of both the proximal and distal divided ends of the vagus.

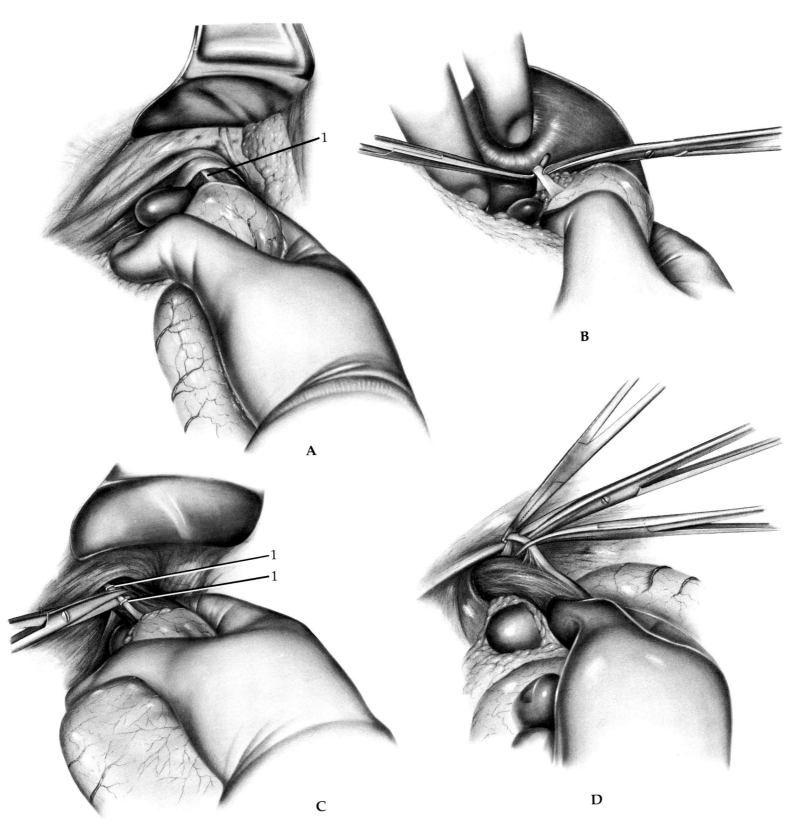

A

B

C

D

13

PLATE 6 • SUBTOTAL GASTRECTOMY — cont'd

A After the vagotomy has been completed, attention is directed to continuing the mobilization of the stomach. The method described subsequently has proved satisfactory and saves a considerable amount of time when compared with the more routinely used method of separating the omentum from the greater curvature of the stomach, a dissection that is frequently bloody, time-consuming, and tedious. The embryology of the omentum is such that it is not attached to the colon in its embryologic development. It becomes an easy matter, therefore, to separate the omentum from the transverse colon. The omentum is first grasped by the left hand (1) of the operating surgeon and the left hand (2) of the first assistant, and tension is developed between the transverse colon (3) and the posterior aspect of the greater omentum (4). The dissection is begun with dissecting scissors, and the plane of dissection is an avascular one.

B Once the dissection has been started and the tissue plane opened, gentle traction downward on the colon with a gauze pad (1) further delineates the area to be subsequently divided.

C After the area has been delineated, gentle traction is maintained inferiorly on the transverse colon and superiorly on the greater omentum, while the dissecting scissors are used to separate the omentum from the transverse colon.

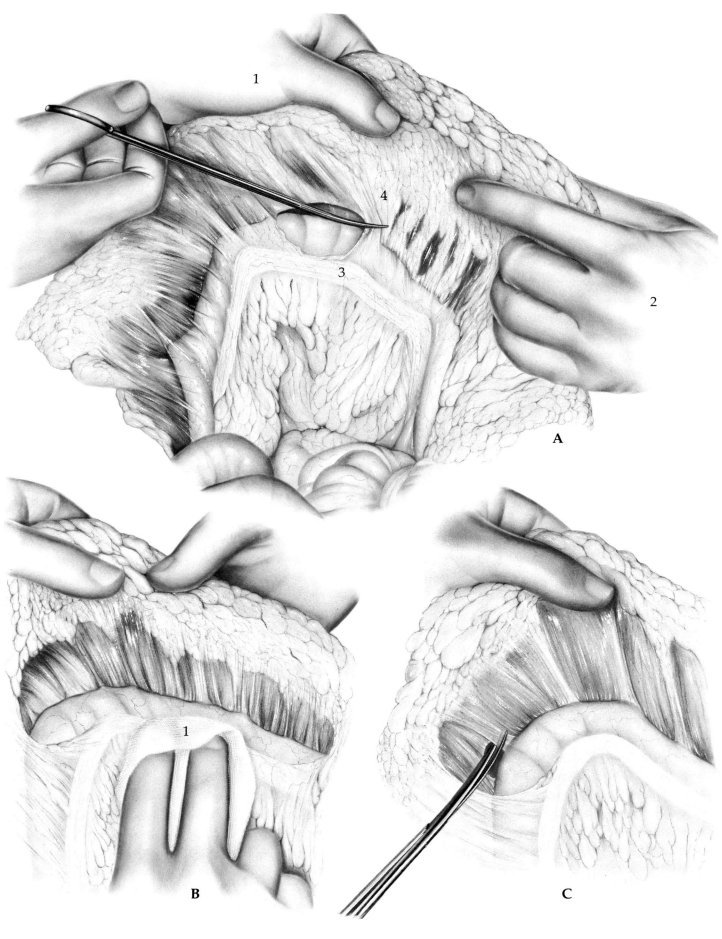

PLATE 7 • SUBTOTAL GASTRECTOMY—cont'd

A Occasionally small vessels are encountered in the course of this dissection and are managed by suture ligation *(1)*. Suture ligatures are preferred to free ties, particularly in areas where the vessel to be dealt with is attached to a hollow viscus. Subsequent distention of a hollow viscus has the potential hazard of extruding the free tie from the divided end of the vessel, allowing for postoperative hemorrhage.

B Further dissection separates the omentum from the transverse colon. Note the proximity of the division of this tissue plane to the colon wall *(1)*. Some care must be exercised here not to injure the colon, but this dissection can be easily accomplished.

C The dissection is continued to the right side of the transverse colon, the stomach *(1)* superiorly and the colon *(2)* inferiorly, with the stomach in the right hand of the first assistant. Note that the dissecting instrument has been changed from the scissors to the knife. The portion of the dissection that comes toward the surgeon is more easily executed with the knife than with the scissors, which require a slightly awkward position.

D The avascularity of this plane of dissection separating the omentum from the transverse colon is apparent.

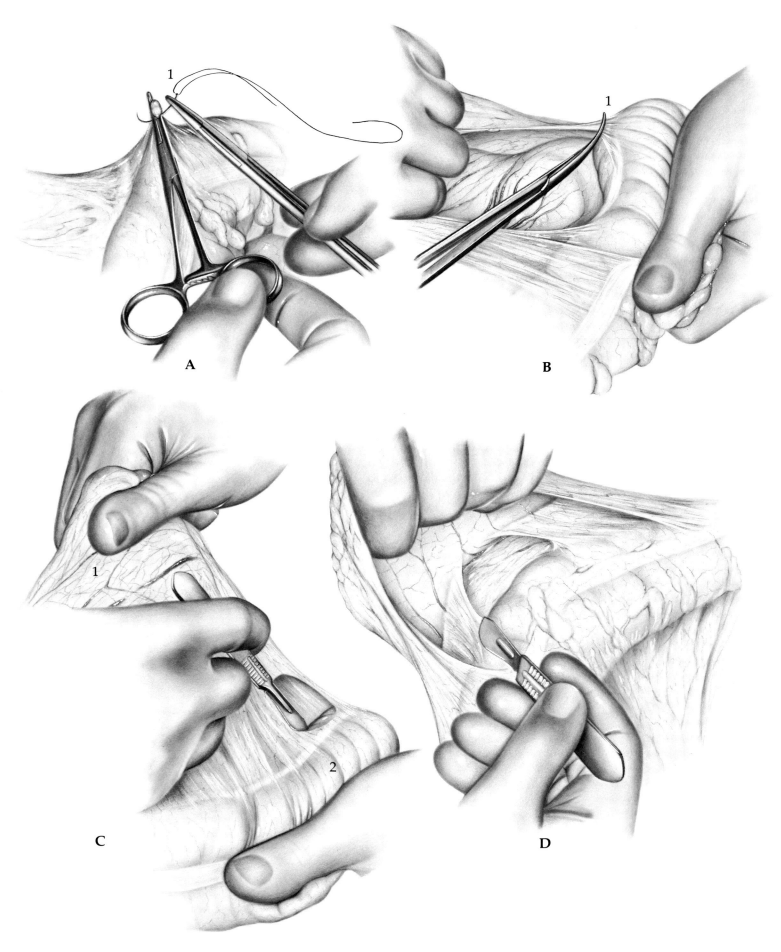

A

B

C

D

PLATE 8 • SUBTOTAL GASTRECTOMY—cont'd

A The omentum (1) and stomach can be seen retracted superiorly and the colon (2) inferiorly; forceps are being used to point out branches of the middle colic artery (3). One advantage of this method of opening the lesser sac is minimizing the risk of injury to the middle colic artery, since the vessel is exposed at the periphery rather than at its origin. Early in the dissection any injury to the vessel that may occur with this method of opening the lesser sac has the advantage of affecting simply a distal branch of the major trunk of the middle colic rather than the trunk at its origin—a hazard that exists when the dissection is performed by dividing the omentum from the greater curvature of the stomach.

B The dissection of the omentum from the transverse colon is continued. This time the stomach is retracted superiorly and to the left, and the transverse colon is pulled ventrally and inferiorly.

C The right lobe of the liver (1) can be seen overlying the distal stomach and duodenum. As the stomach is retracted superiorly, the transverse colon now has been dropped out of the operative field underneath the hand tenting the tissue (2), between the stomach and the pancreas posteriorly.

D A continuation of this dissection is shown toward the lesser curvature (1). Again for reorientation the stomach and omentum are in the hand retracting the stomach superiorly (2). The pancreas (3) can be seen lying transversely across the operative field, and the transverse colon (4) is depressed by the assistant's hand. Several filmy adhesions (5) are usually present between the posterior gastric wall and the anterior surface of the pancreas. These again are avascular and may be divided with safety.

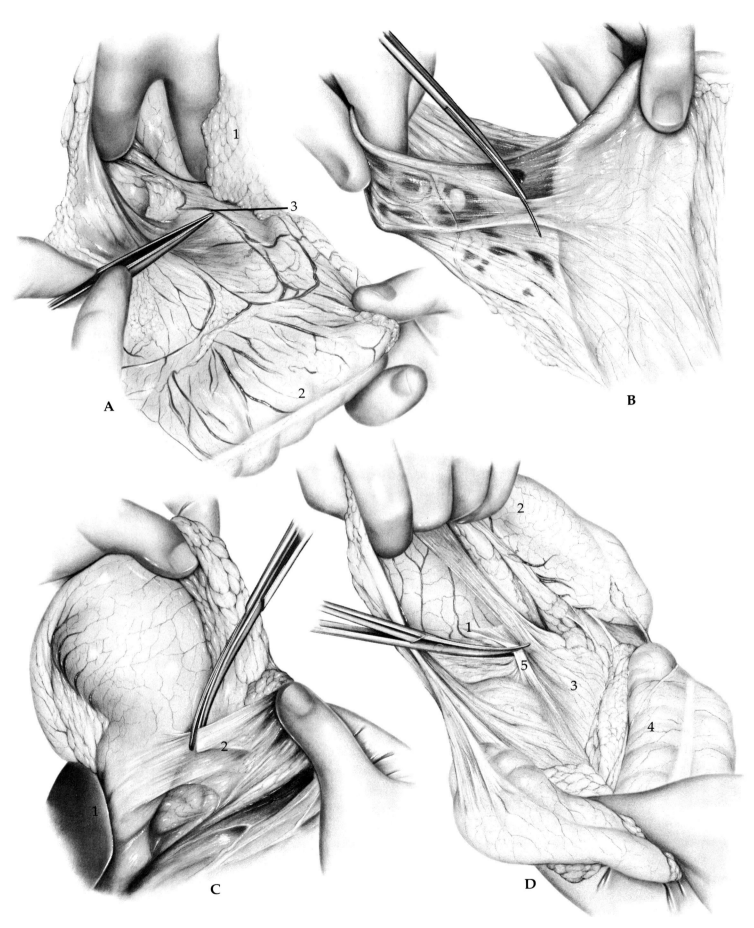

A

B

C

D

19

PLATE 9 • SUBTOTAL GASTRECTOMY — cont'd

A The stomach *(1)* is retracted superiorly in the surgeon's left hand, and the transverse colon *(2)* is retracted inferiorly in the surgeon's right hand, with the index fingers of each hand used to separate the filmy areolar tissue connecting the omentum to the right portion of the anterior surface of the pancreas *(3)*. This again is generally an avascular plane of dissection, but the finger dissection should be carried out with some gentleness, since occasionally veins in this area may be torn, resulting in bothersome but not serious hemorrhage.

B Once this area of the dissection has been completed, the only remaining attachment between the omentum and the transverse colon is a portion *(1)* that runs down toward the superior aspect of the hepatic flexure. This is shown, between the right and left hands of the surgeon, being held up ready for clamping, division, and suture ligature. This final step completes the mobilization of the greater curvature of the stomach from the other intra-abdominal organs, notably the pancreas and transverse colon.

C The beginning of the Kocher maneuver is shown. Babcock clamps have been placed on the descending portion of the duodenum *(1)*, and the duodenum has been retracted medially. The right lobe of the liver *(2)* can be seen held out of the way with a Richardson retractor. A Deaver retractor *(3)* is placed in the inferior aspect of the abdominal wound. By retracting the duodenum medially, the tissue plane between the duodenum and the lateral peritoneum can be easily identified. This lateral peritoneal reflection is also an avascular plane. This plane is shown being entered with the tissue forceps tenting up the tissue, and the tissue scissors are being used to divide or enter the area lateral to the duodenum. Once a 1.5 cm. incision is made in this area, the remainder of the dissection is carried out by using the surgeon's index fingers.

D The performance of this blunt dissection is shown with the duodenum retracted medially and with the index fingers used to gently but bluntly open up the retro-duodenal area. The vena cava *(1)* is exposed with this maneuver and is without danger of being injured because of the blunt nature of the dissection. After this tissue plane has been opened, the surgeon can easily insert his examining hand posterior to the duodenum and then perform a bimanual examination of the duodenum and the head of the pancreas. The previous separation of the omentum from this area allows this examination to be accomplished with no interference from other tissue.

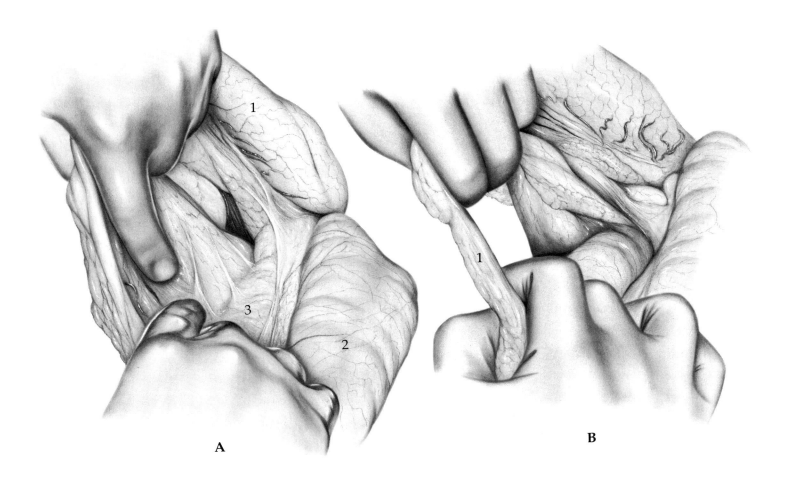

A

B

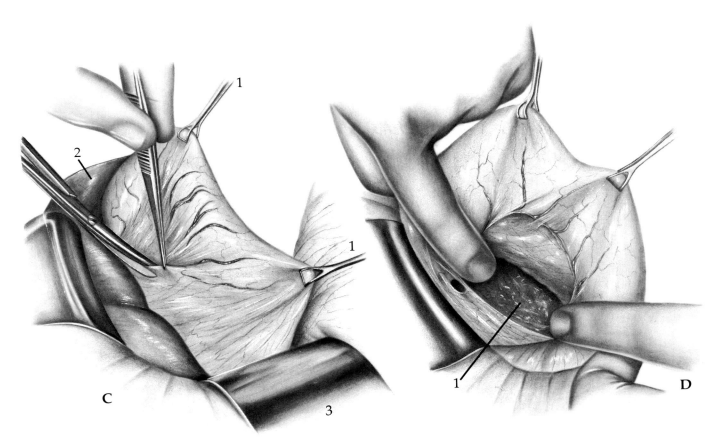

C

D

21

PLATE 10 • SUBTOTAL GASTRECTOMY — cont'd

After the stomach has been freed of its inferior attachments by dissection of the omentum and the Kocher maneuver has been performed, the mobilization of the stomach is continued.

A This step demonstrates the management of the right gastroepiploic vessels. It will be noted that there are three *(1, 2, 3)* hemostats placed on the epiploic pedicle; the dissecting scissors *(4)* are then used to divide the pedicle between hemostats 1 and 2. A free 2-0 silk ligature is then placed underneath clamp 3. Clamp 3 is removed and the ligature is tightened. A suture of 3-0 silk is then placed between the first free tie and clamp 2, and the pedicle is doubly ligated with the suture ligature. Clamp 1 is ligated with a 2-0 free tie after division of the epiploic pedicle has been accomplished.

B Additional freedom of the proximal duodenum *(1)* is accomplished by division of this epiploic pedicle *(2)*, once the previously described posterior dissection of the stomach has been completed.

C Attention is now directed to the right gastric artery. By elevating the stomach ventrally, the right gastric pedicle is stretched tightly, and the right gastric artery is brought into close approximation to the stomach. This important feature avoids injury to the gastroduodenal artery. With the left hand *(1)* placed behind the right gastric pedicle, a sharp right-angle clamp is introduced at the lesser curvature aspect of the gastroduodenal junction, and by using the left hand to control the tip of the instrument, the right gastric artery is isolated. The management of the right gastric artery is accomplished in a fashion similar to that for the gastroepiploic pedicle.

D After the right gastric artery has been divided *(1)* between hemostats and the proximal end suture ligated, the gastroduodenal junction is found to be free from its posterior, superior, and inferior attachments.

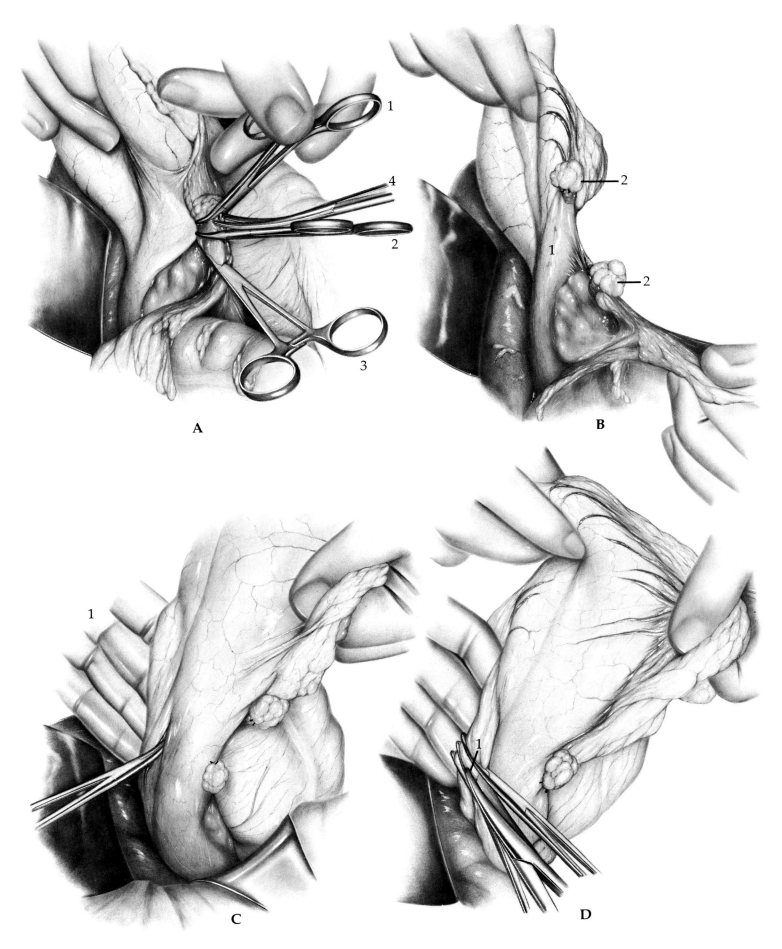

A

B

C

D

PLATE 11 • SUBTOTAL GASTRECTOMY — cont'd

A With the stomach now retracted superiorly, exposing the posterior portion of the gastroduodenal junction, fine Halsted hemostats are used; the tissue between the posterior aspect of the proximal duodenum (1) and the head of the pancreas (2) is carefully dissected free, and each small vessel suture is ligated.

B Notice that the hemostats (1) are placed only on the tissue on the pancreatic side, since there is little bleeding from the gastric side.

C Suture ligation of these vessels is important for two reasons: first, to avoid excessive injury to the pancreas and, second, because small bites of tissue are much more easily controlled with suture ligatures than they are with free ties.

D A portion of the duodenum (1) has been freed from its attachment to the pancreas. It is an important consideration at this point to note that only a short portion of the duodenum is separated from the pancreas. The duodenal blood supply is sparse, and it is important not to have an excess of duodenum dissected from its blood supply, which comes from vessels shared by the duodenum and the pancreas in this area. After this dissection has been accomplished, the duodenum is then free and a noncrushing vascular clamp (2) is placed across the duodenum. A second clamp, which may be of a crushing type (3) (a Kocher is suitable), is then placed on the stomach side of the duodenum at this point, and the tissue between the two clamps is divided with a scalpel. Note that about 2 mm. of duodenum (4) is allowed to extend beyond the noncrushing clamp. This maneuver prevents slippage of the duodenum from the jaws of this clamp as the remainder of the operation is completed.

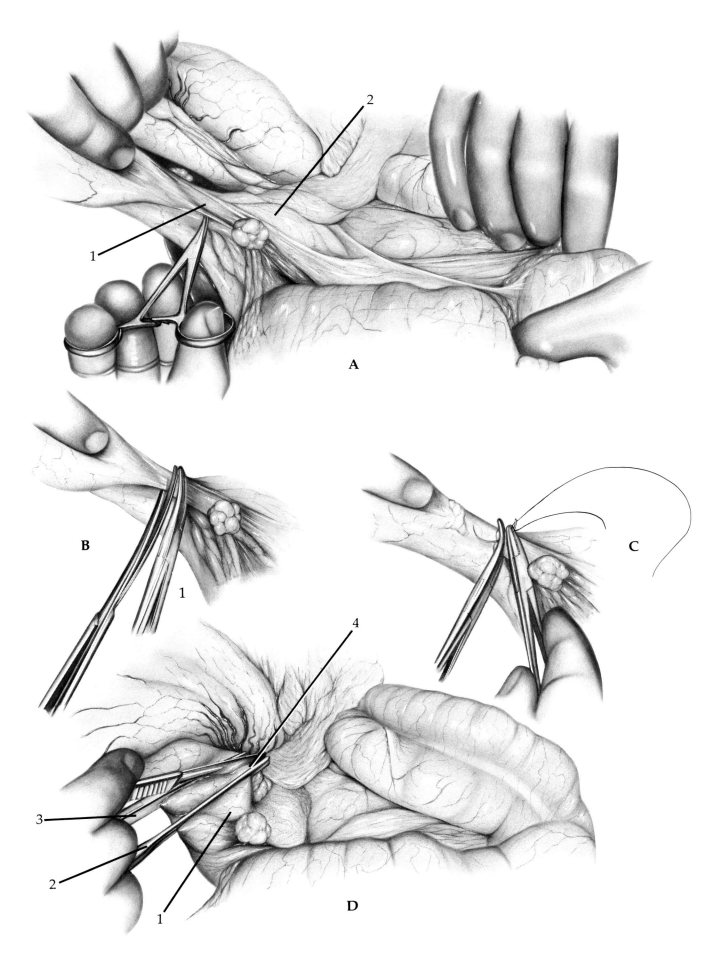

A

B

C

D

1

2

3

4

25

PLATE 12 • SUBTOTAL GASTRECTOMY — cont'd

A After the stomach has been divided from the duodenum, the crushing clamp *(1)* on the duodenum can now be used to pull the stomach toward the patient's right, and the surgeon then inspects the stomach and selects the area for gastric resection. On the lesser curvature the veins entering the lesser curvature of the stomach are identified, and the third vein *(2)* from the gastroesophageal junction is selected for site of division on the lesser curvature aspect of the stomach. As the greater curvature area is inspected, a point at which the gastroepiploic vessels seem to come closest to the stomach *(3)* is selected for the division of the stomach on the greater curvature side.

B After *A* has been accomplished, the omentum is now divided *(1)* from its free edge inferiorly up toward the greater curvature of the stomach. By flattening the omentum the blood vessels can be readily identified and precisely clamped with small, curved Halsted clamps. Those vessels on the portion of stomach to remain are managed with suture ligatures, and those on the specimen are simply tied. This can often be accomplished with only one or two hemostats if the surgeon is careful in inspecting the omentum and in choosing a plane of minimal vascularity through which to divide the greater omentum. As the omentum is divided in a perpendicular fashion toward the greater curvature of the stomach, the last vessel to be encountered will be a branch of the epiploic system.

C A hemostat *(1)* is being introduced from the inferior aspect of the omentum at the edge of the greater curvature of the stomach, and the remaining gastroepiploic vessel is divided at this point. Hemostats can be identified *(2, 3)* on the divided omentum. Hemostat 2 is on the portion of the omentum to be removed with the specimen, and hemostat 3 is on the portion of the omentum that will remain. It is preferable to resect the omentum attached to the portion of stomach removed en bloc with the specimen. This method is chosen to avoid excessive amounts of omentum with marginal blood supply remaining with the gastric remnant. In addition, a large mass of omentum results in significant added weight to the gastric remnant, which tends to put disruptive force on the gastroduodenal anastomosis.

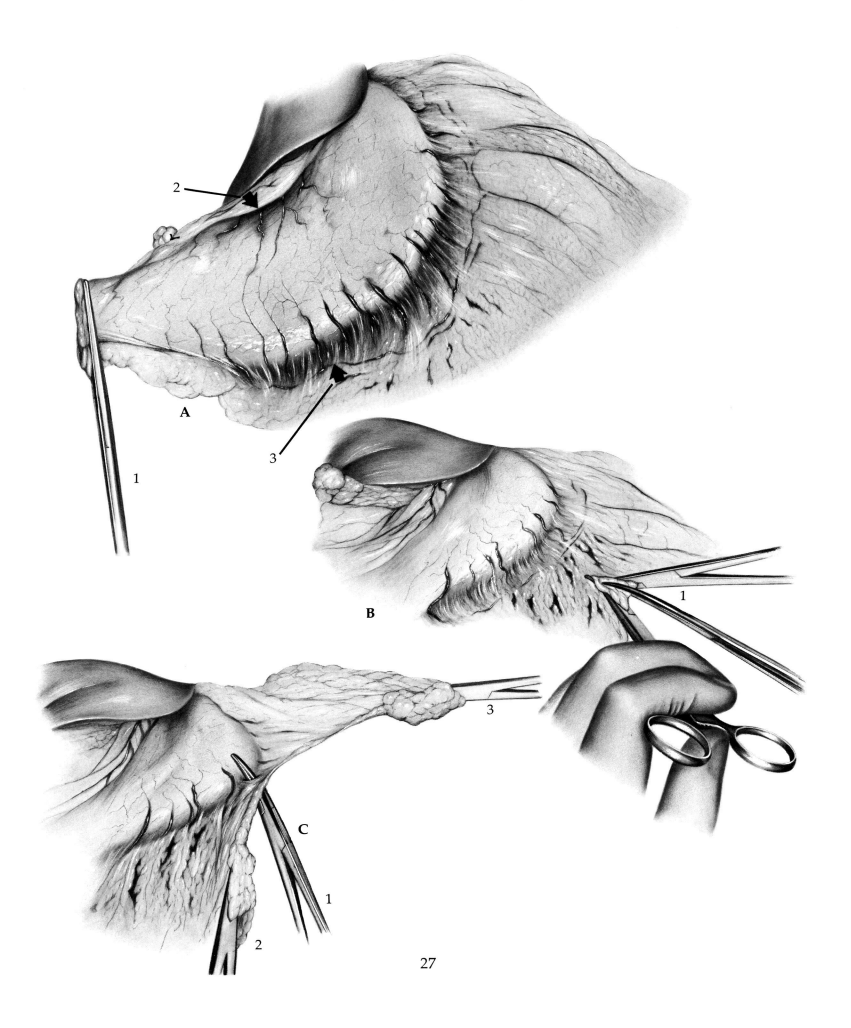

A

B

C

PLATE 13 • SUBTOTAL GASTRECTOMY — cont'd

A After the final bit of omental tissue has been separated from the greater curvature of the stomach, this tissue is isolated between hemostats and divided with the scissors. The portion remaining with the stomach *(1)* is suture ligated, and the portion resected *(2)* is tied.

B An area of approximately 2½ inches of greater curvature has been entirely dissected free of omental attachments, and three stay sutures *(1, 2, 3)* have been placed. For these stay sutures 3-0 silk is satisfactory, and they are placed approximately one fingerbreadth apart. The area of gastric resection will be between sutures 2 and 3. Suture 1 remains on the corner of what will subsequently be the gastroduodenal anastomosis.

C Attention is now directed to the lesser curvature of the stomach. A hemostat directs attention to the site of resection *(1)* on the lesser curvature as previously described (Plate 12, *A*).

D The lesser omentum is separated from the lesser curvature of the stomach and divided between hemostats. Care must be taken to execute this dissection close to the gastric wall to avoid injury to the hepatic artery.

E The dissection in the lesser omentum continues into the posterior leaf of the lesser omentum. Once the lesser omentum has been freed from the lesser curvature of the stomach, it will be obvious that the lesser curvature has an area of approximately 0.5 cm. in width that is not covered with peritoneum. This results from the anatomic manner in which the lesser omentum is attached to the lesser curvature.

F Three stay sutures are placed approximately a fingerbreadth apart, and they are placed in a manner so as to approximate the peritoneum over the anterior and posterior gastric walls, recovering the lesser curvature with peritoneum at the site of intended anastomosis.

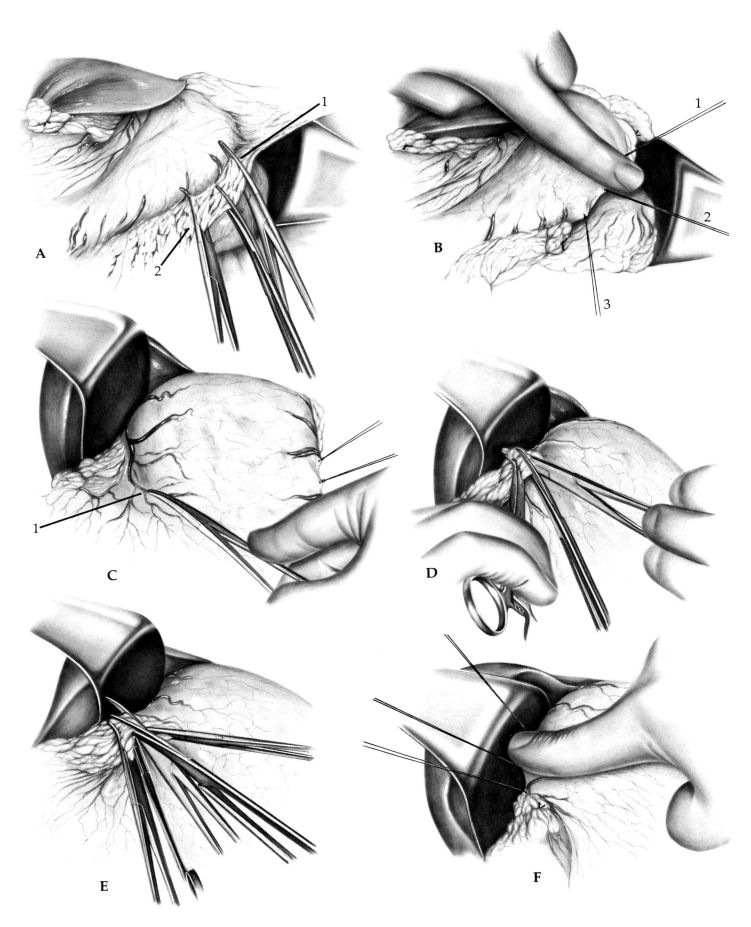

PLATE 14 • SUBTOTAL GASTRECTOMY — cont'd

A A crushing Payr clamp *(1)* is placed across the full width of the stomach between the middle and distal stay sutures. Note that on the lesser curvature the peritoneum *(2)* has been reapproximated over the bare portion of the stomach. This Payr clamp is then closed, crushing the stomach at the intended site of resection. Prior to closing the clamp it is wise for the surgeon to carefully palpate for the nasogastric tube to be certain that the tube is not included in the clamp.

B The stomach is gathered into a small cylinder for the placement of the VonPetz sewing clamp *(1)*. The VonPetz clamp is then placed across the stomach at the site from which the Payr clamp has been removed. Prior to the closing of the VonPetz clamp, traction is placed on the stomach distally and care is taken not to flatten the stomach prior to closing the VonPetz clamp.

C The securing ring clamp *(1)* is placed over the end of the VonPetz clamp, and the handle *(2)* turned clockwise to insert a double row of silver staples.

D The staples *(1)* hemostatically approximate the anterior and posterior gastric walls and leave a bridge of tissue 1.5 cm. in width that has been crushed between the two rows of staples.

E The placement of the Von Haberer sutures is the next step in the gastrectomy. This part of the procedure is of critical importance, since it allows the end-to-end approximation of the stomach to the duodenum and eliminates the usual lesser curvature closure. French-eye needles are used with 3-0 interrupted silk, and the sutures are placed 1 cm. proximal to the first row of VonPetz staples. These sutures are taken through the full thickness of the stomach, transfixing the mucosa to the gastric wall so that it neither retracts nor protrudes after the stomach has been divided. Moderately large bites of stomach are taken, utilizing about six sutures in the anterior and six in the posterior wall of the stomach.

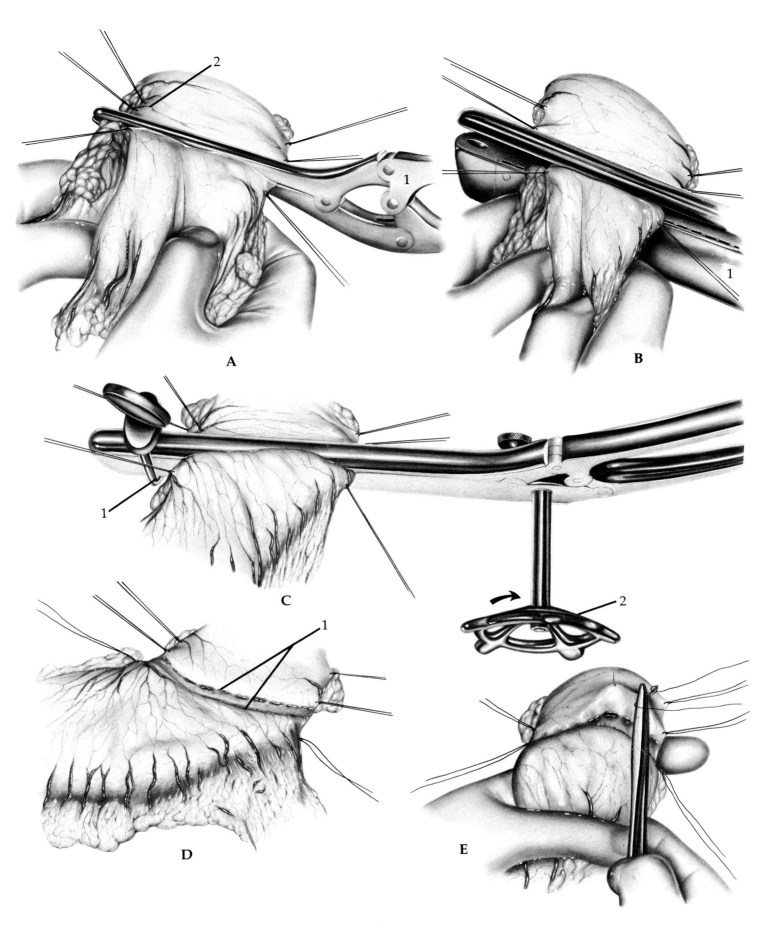

A

B

C

D

E

31

PLATE 15 • SUBTOTAL GASTRECTOMY — cont'd

A The anterior row of Von Haberer sutures has been placed and tied in this example; seven sutures were required across the anterior aspect of the stomach. Constant tension is applied to the portion of the stomach *(1)* to be resected in order to keep the gastric remnant narrowed.

B After the anterior row of sutures has been completed, the distal stomach is elevated, exposing the posterior gastric wall, and the posterior row of Von Haberer sutures is inserted.

C The posterior Von Haberer sutures have been placed and tied. Note again that there is approximately 1 cm. *(1)* of distance between the Von Haberer sutures and the first row of VonPetz staples.

D The anterior portion of the stomach is divided with a scalpel between the VonPetz staples and the Von Haberer sutures. This maneuver can be accomplished either with a scalpel or with the heavy scissors.

E The gastric division has been completed, with the gastric stoma having been narrowed. Note that the mucosa has been transfixed to the full thickness of the stomach wall.

F The gastric opening now admits only two fingers.

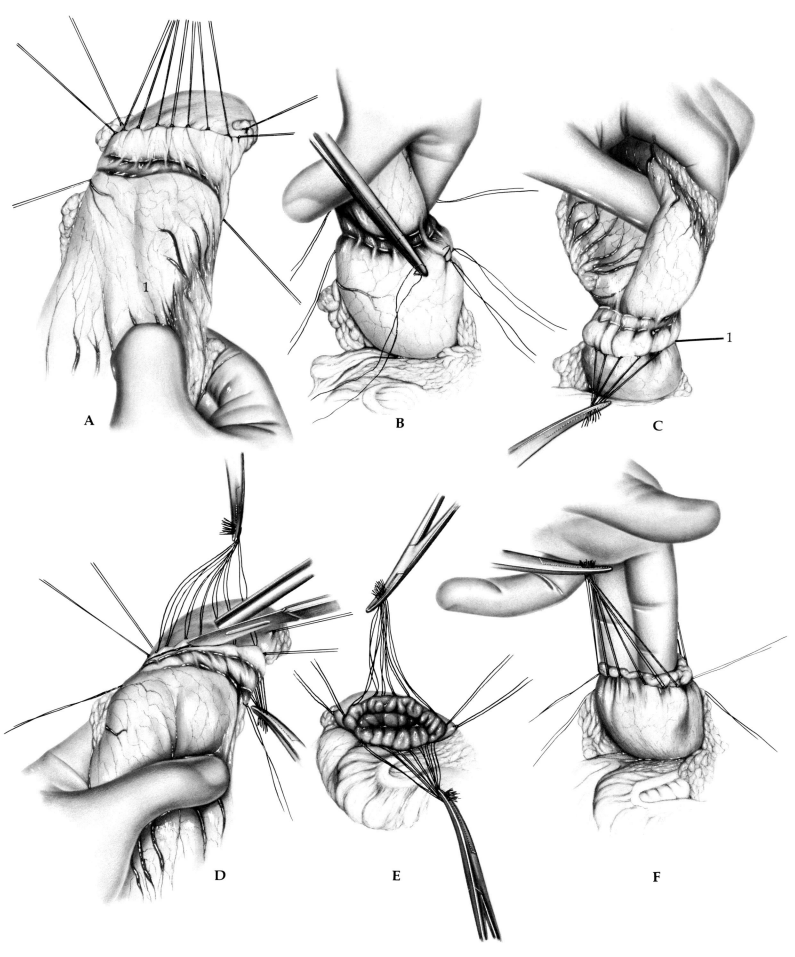

PLATE 16 • GASTRODUODENOSTOMY, BILLROTH I PRINCIPLE

A By placing traction on the posterior row of Von Haberer sutures *(1)*, the stomach is easily pulled down to the duodenum *(2)*, which is seen held in the noncrushing clamp. This maneuver is accomplished without tension. Absence of tension is the direct result of the previously described mobilization of the stomach.

B Here the corner suture *(1)* has been inserted between the lesser curvature of the stomach and the lesser curvature aspect of the duodenum.

C The posterior row of the gastroduodenostomy is continued. Mattress sutures *(1)* of 3-0 silk are placed between the posterior gastric wall and the posterior duodenal wall, and are left untied until completion of the suture line.

D The second suture *(1)* in the posterior row of the gastroduodenostomy is shown. The Von Haberer sutures *(2)* are useful in applying traction to expose the posterior aspect of the stomach.

E As the suture line is continued across the posterior stomach and duodenum, the sutures are placed in the stomach just proximal *(1)* to the Von Haberer sutures. If the duodenum and the stomach have been properly mobilized, the anastomosis is carried out with excellent exposure even in obese patients. Again the key to the execution of this portion of the operation is adequate previous mobilization of both the stomach and the duodenum.

F Notice in the placement of this row of sutures that the bite taken on the stomach exceeds the size of that taken on the duodenum. This technique further eliminates the despairity between the gastric and the duodenal stomal sizes.

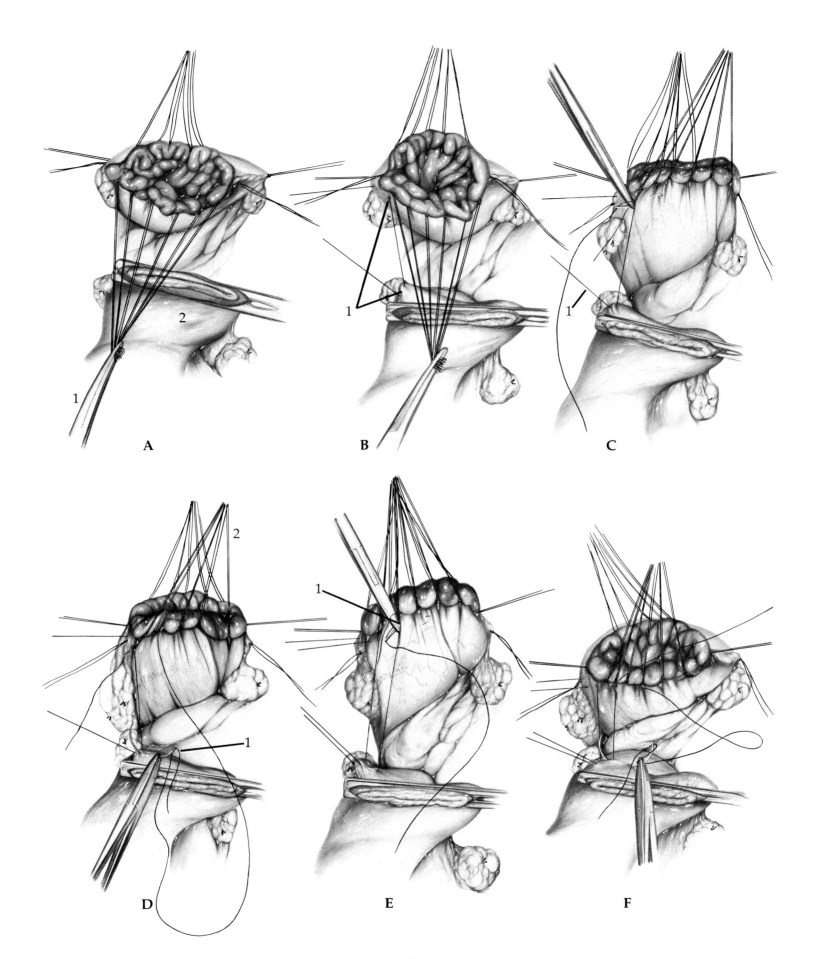

A   B   C

D   E   F

35

PLATE 17 • GASTRODUODENOSTOMY, BILLROTH I PRINCIPLE—cont'd

A to C As the posterior seromuscular row of sutures is continued, notice the importance of not only the greater size of the bites taken on the gastric wall but also the greater distance between the sutures on the gastric side and then the duodenal side. This again assists in elimination of despairity between the gastric and duodenal stomas.

D to F As the posterior seromuscular row nears completion, it can be appreciated that the stomach and duodenum are going to be easily approximated in an end-to-end fashion. The final suture *(1)* depicted in *F* indicates the importance of encompassing the full thickness of the duodenum and stomach at the corner to provide added security at this important point. Note that on the gastric side the needle has been introduced on the posterior aspect of the stomach and is exiting on the anterior aspect; the needle being inserted into the anterior aspect of the duodenum and exiting on the posterior aspect provides the added security at this crucial point in the anastomotic completion.

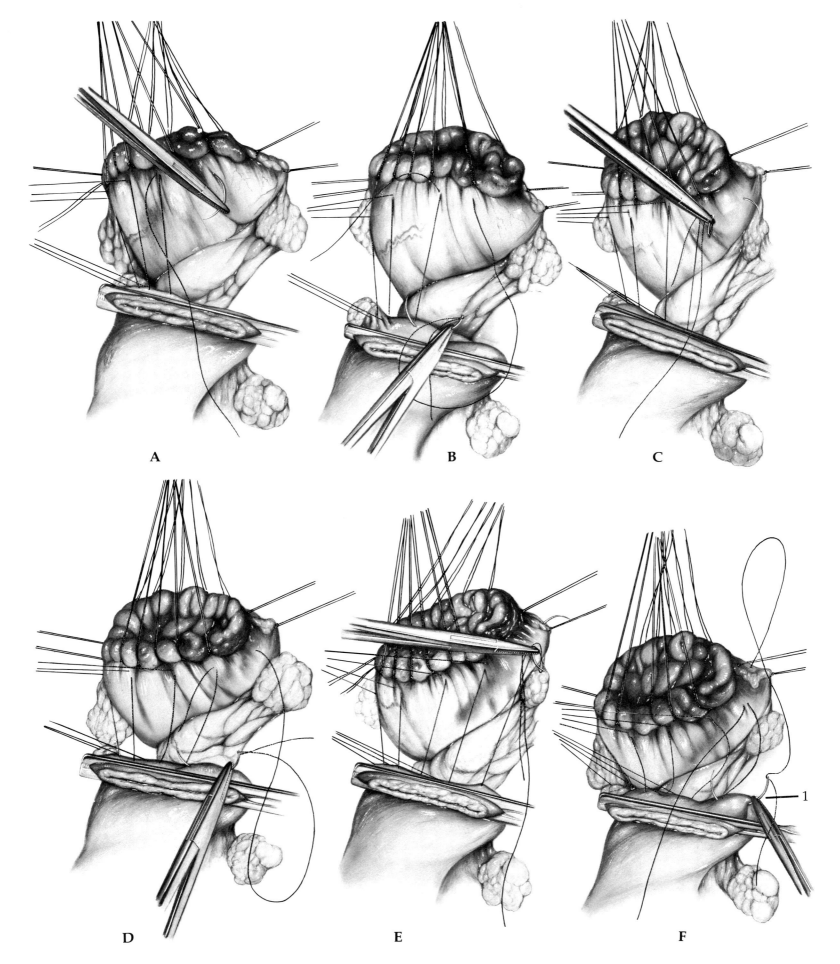

A

B

C

D

E

F

1

PLATE 18 • GASTRODUODENOSTOMY, BILLROTH I PRINCIPLE — cont'd

A The anterior seromuscular portion of the anastomosis is begun. The suture *(1)* is inserted into the stomach at the site of omental attachment to the greater curvature and exits on the anterior gastric wall.

B The noncrushing clamp is now turned, exposing the anterior surface of the duodenum *(1)*. The suture is inserted into the anterior aspect of the duodenum and exits at exactly the corner of the anastomosis.

C The corner stitch *(1)* on the greater curvature has been tied. The remaining posterior seromuscular sutures are now tied with the noncrushing clamp still on the duodenum.

D The corner suture *(1)* on the lesser curvature aspect of the anastomosis is identified. The posterior seromuscular row of sutures has now been completed.

E The posterior seromuscular sutures are left intact while the posterior Von Haberer *(1)* sutures are now being cut.

F After dividing the Von Haberer sutures, the noncrushing clamp is removed from the duodenum, and the surgeon is now prepared to begin the mucosa-to-mucosa approximation of the posterior row.

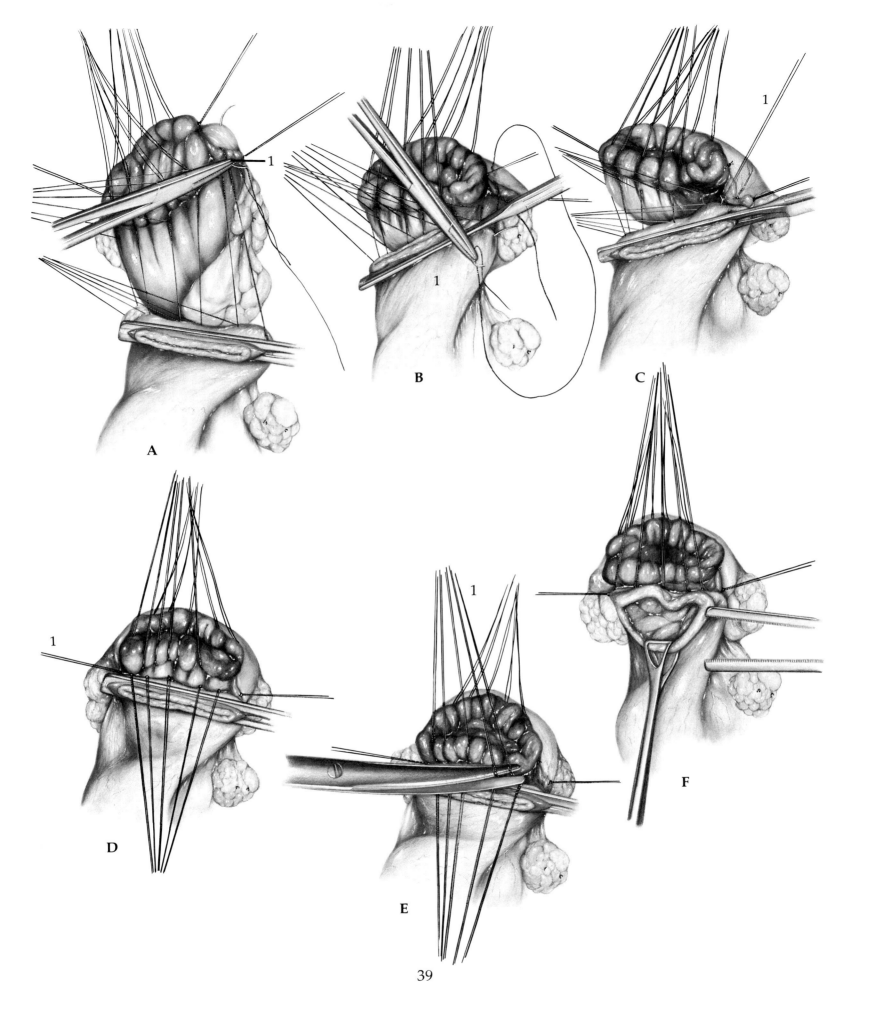

PLATE 19 • GASTRODUODENOSTOMY, BILLROTH I PRINCIPLE — cont'd

A With the seromuscular sutures *(1)* still uncut, the first suture *(2)* is placed in the mucosa-to-mucosa approximation. Note the clamp *(3)* on the anterior rim of the duodenum that facilitates exposure of the anastomosis.

B A seromuscular suture is being cut after the first mucosa-to-mucosa suture *(1)* has been inserted, but before it is tied.

C This technique is carried out across the entire posterior row of the anastomosis and greatly facilitates the accuracy of the placement of the mucosa-to-mucosa approximating stitches.

D The entire mucosa-to-mucosa posterior layer has been inserted, and the sutures are now being cut.

E The next step in the anastomosis is the cutting of the Von Haberer sutures on the anterior wall of the stomach.

F Beginning on the lesser curvature side of the stomach, the anterior inverting row of mucosa-approximating sutures is begun. This is done in an interrupted Connell fashion. Beginning just at the corner of the internal aspect of the duodenum *(1)*, a 3-0 silk suture on a French-eye needle is inserted from within the duodenum through the full thickness to the outside.

G The needle is now withdrawn from within the gastric lumen, creating inversion at the corner of the lesser curvature aspect of the anastomosis.

H The suture having been inserted, gentle back-and-forth traction is placed on it to assist in the inversion.

I If this gentle back-and-forth sawing motion is not effective at causing inversion, the inversion can be assisted by gentle pressure with a gauze sponge over the index finger of the first assistant.

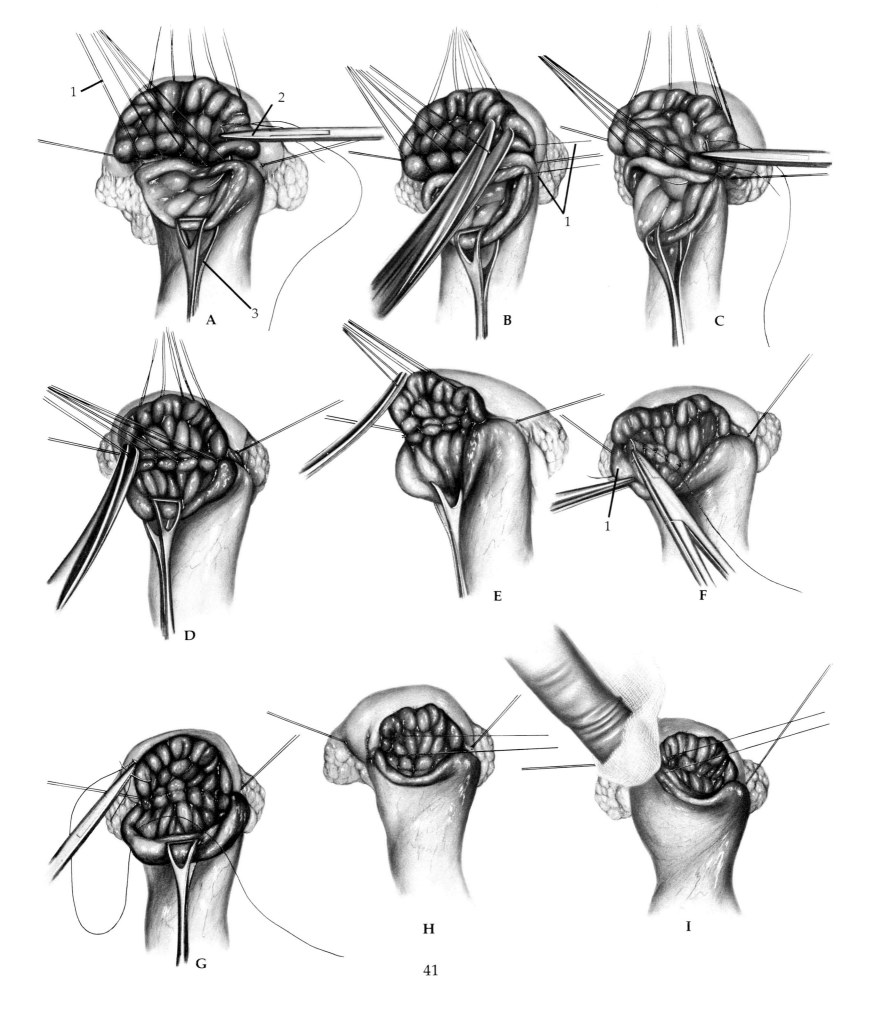

PLATE 20 • GASTRODUODENOSTOMY, BILLROTH I PRINCIPLE—cont'd

A After inversion of the lesser curvature aspect of the anastomosis has been accomplished, attention is directed to the greater curvature aspect.

B The insertion of this row of sutures from the two corners of the anastomosis toward the center is shown.

C Note the ease with which inversion is accomplished.

D The next to last anterior suture is inserted.

E The final suture is being placed. The previous suture *(1)* has been left untied.

F Forceps are used to assist with inversion as the final two sutures are tied.

G The suture line has been completed, with the final two Connell sutures having been tied. The only step remaining for the completion of the gastroduodenostomy is the placement of the anterior seromuscular sutures.

H This row of stitches is quite important in this method of anastomosis and takes advantage of the fact that the gastric circumference exceeds the duodenal circumference a short distance from the previously placed inverting suture line. The first anterior seromuscular suture has been inserted through the gastric wall at the lesser curvature corner of the anastomosis.

I The stitch can be seen inserted into the duodenal wall, and the insertion of the needle into the duodenum is not opposite the exit site from the stomach. This is intentional and the duodenal suture should be considered as the apex of a triangle that will have its base on the gastric wall.

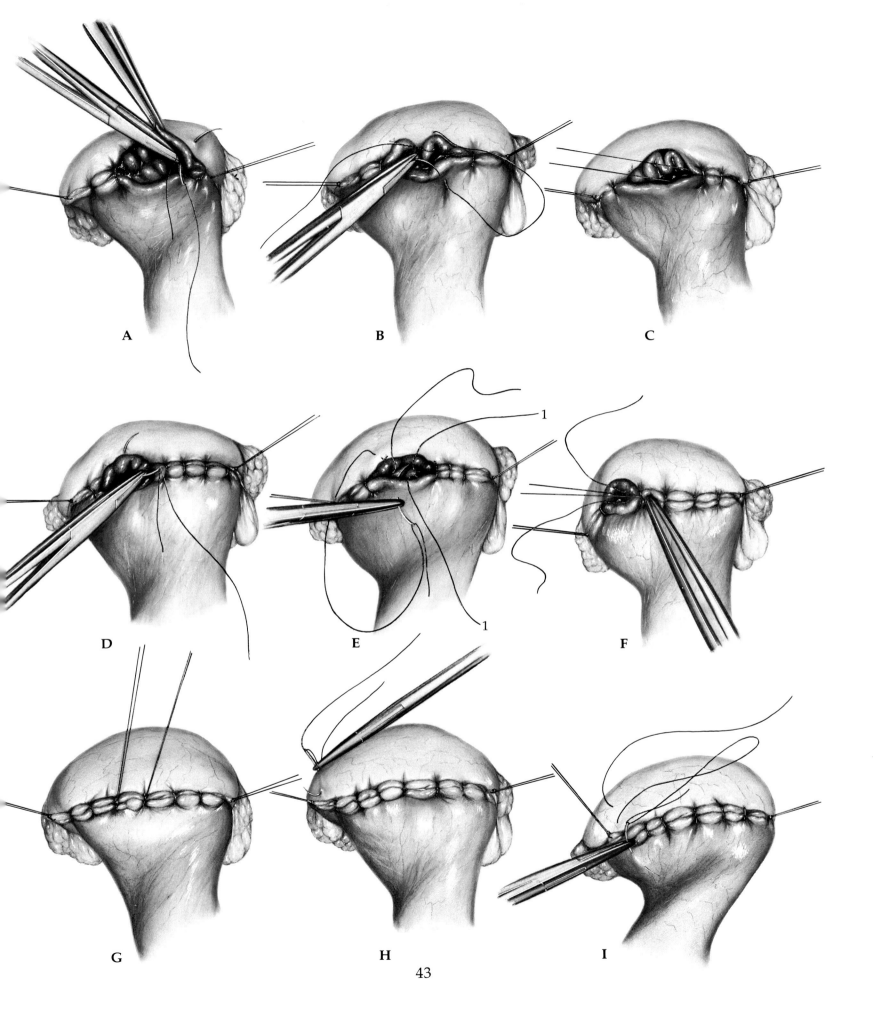

A   B   C

D   E   F

G   H   I

43

PLATE 21 • GASTRODUODENOSTOMY, BILLROTH I PRINCIPLE—cont'd

A The placement of the third portion of the seromuscular suture establishes the equilateral triangle, with its base on the stomach and its apex on the duodenum. With slight upward traction the stomach wall is telescoped over the previous Connell suture line; this method of suture placement avoids the potential narrowing of the duodenal lumen. Each of these stitches is tied after its placement.

B The first suture is ready for tying.

C After the first two sutures have been placed, care must be taken that the needle exits on the stomach side of the anastomosis just at the previously performed Connell suture line *(1)*. This avoids excessive tissue being rolled into the anastomosis.

D The concept of using the duodenal suture as the apex of an equilateral triangle is shown.

E Its base is again demonstrated in the placement of the suture on the gastric wall.

F The second bite into the gastric wall is completed and the suture is ready for tying.

G Note that the stomach is pulled down over the gastroduodenal anastomosis, sealing it quite securely.

H The final corner suture is placed, with the previously tagged corner stitch *(1)* being pulled across the anastomotic line to assist in securing adequate inversion of the critical corner.

I After the placement of the final corner stitch, the previous corner stitch *(1)* is divided prior to tying the final corner suture *(2)*.

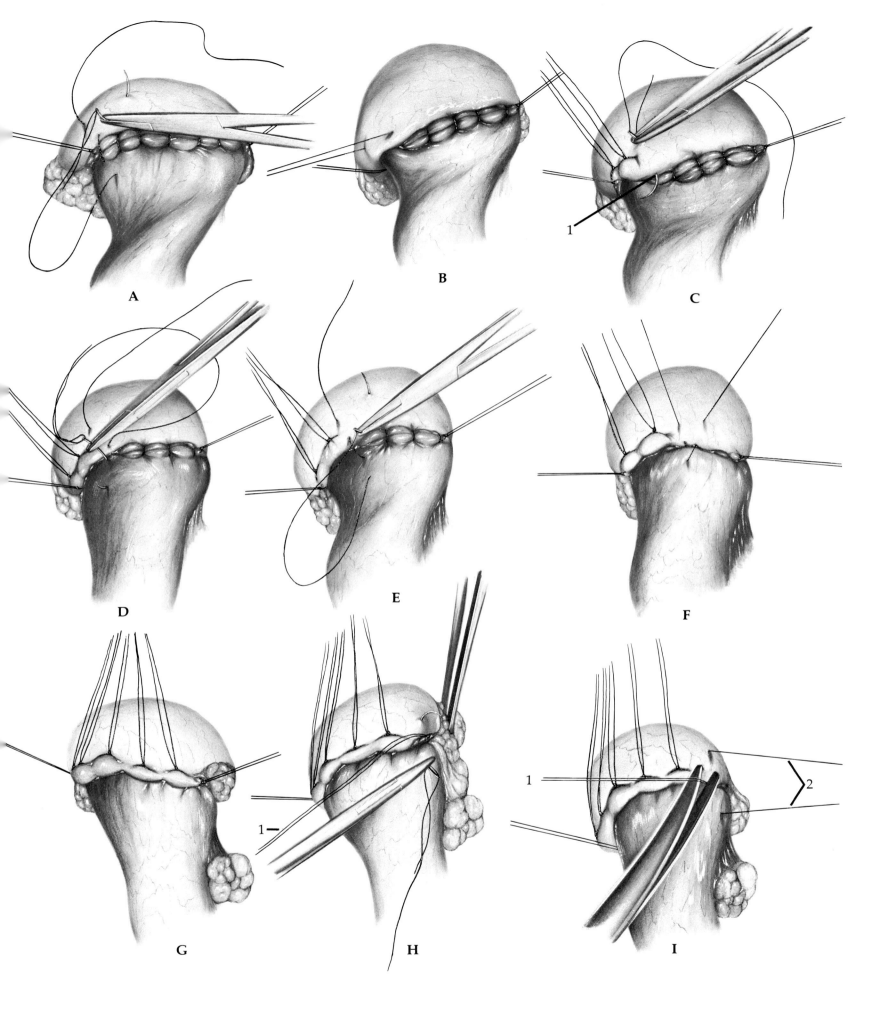

A

B

C

D

E

F

1

G

H

1

I

1

2

PLATE 22 • GASTRODUODENOSTOMY, BILLROTH I PRINCIPLE—cont'd

A The entire seromuscular anastomosis is now complete.

B The sutures are being cut.

C After completion of the anastomosis the surgeon assures himself of its patency by examining it with his thumb and index finger. Ordinarily, the anastomosis will freely admit the thumb from the duodenal side.

D The final security of the anastomosis is provided by suturing the divided gastro-epiploic pedicle stumps *(1)* to further lessen potential tension on the suture line in the event that gastric distention should occur in the early postoperative period.

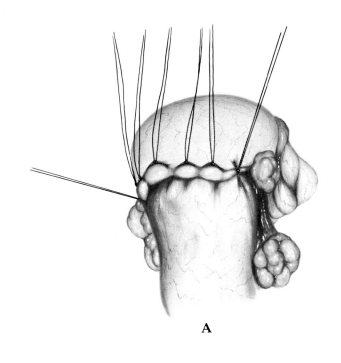

A

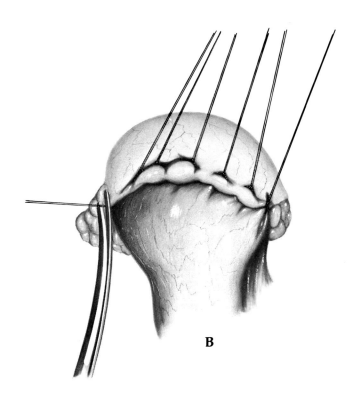

B

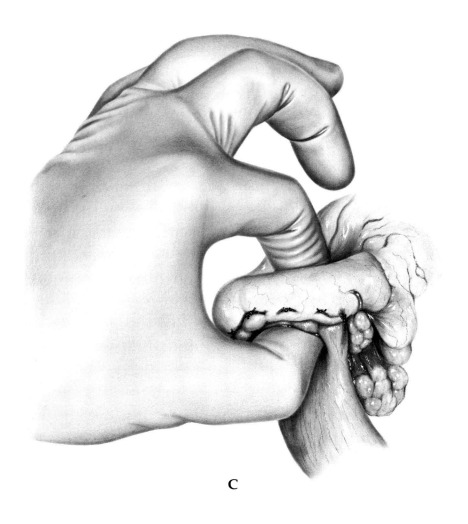

C

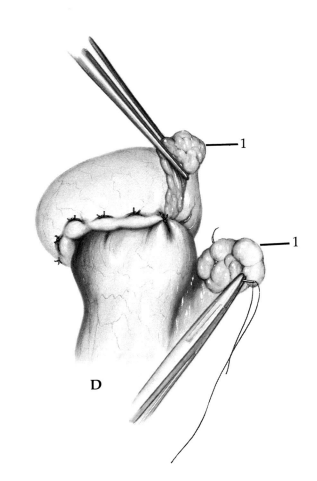

1

1

D

47

CHAPTER
3

Subtotal gastrectomy-gastrojejunostomy

Subtotal gastrectomy with Billroth II gastroenterostomy may be employed with or without vagotomy under specific circumstances.

Since mobilization of the stomach and duodenum is carefully described elsewhere, this will not be repeated. After mobilization of the stomach and duodenum, an Allen clamp is placed across the duodenum just beyond the pylorus. Adequate but not overzealous mobilization is necessary to provide a double suture line and to avoid devascularization of the duodenal stump. An inverting running catgut suture, preferably a double row, with an outer row of inverting silk sutures is employed, and a multiplicity of tissue conserving methods has been described for the difficult duodenal stump. A small (No. 10 French) catheter may be placed through a worrisome suture line into the third portion of the duodenum and brought out, since a duodenostomy is a recommended procedure for the "difficult stump." The preferred method for duodenal stump closure is described in Chapter 8.

PLATE 23 • GASTROJEJUNOSTOMY, BILLROTH II PRINCIPLE, MODIFIED POLYA METHOD

A After the duodenum has been closed, the stomach mobilized, and stay sutures placed on the gastric pouch, the VonPetz clamp is utilized to place a double row of silver staples across the stomach. The position of the gastric tube is checked prior to this step. The point of placement of the clamp may range from the level of the esophagogastric junction on the lesser curvature to the midpoint of the lesser curvature, depending on the size of the remaining gastric pouch desired for specific indications.

B The stomach is divided between rows of staples.

C With traction on Allis clamps *(1)* placed distal to the staples on the cut gastric edge, a partial closure along the lesser curvature is carried out, employing a double row of inverting continuous catgut sutures *(2)*, reenforced with an outer layer of inverting, interrupted silk *(3)*.

D The cut gastric edge held in the Allis clamps is 2 inches long at this point and becomes narrower with subsequent suturing. The corner silk is used for traction *(1)*.

E The gastric pouch is drawn through a 2-inch opening *(1)* in an avascular portion of the transverse colon mesentery to the left of the middle colic vessels and at the midpoint between the transverse colon and the origin of its mesentery.

F The posterior edge of the opening in the mesentery is sutured to the gastric pouch 1 inch from the stapled edge. This avoids the difficult exposure required to close the defect in the mesentery after completion of the anastomosis. After completion of this suture line, corner sutures *(1)* for outlining the gastrojejunostomy are inserted.

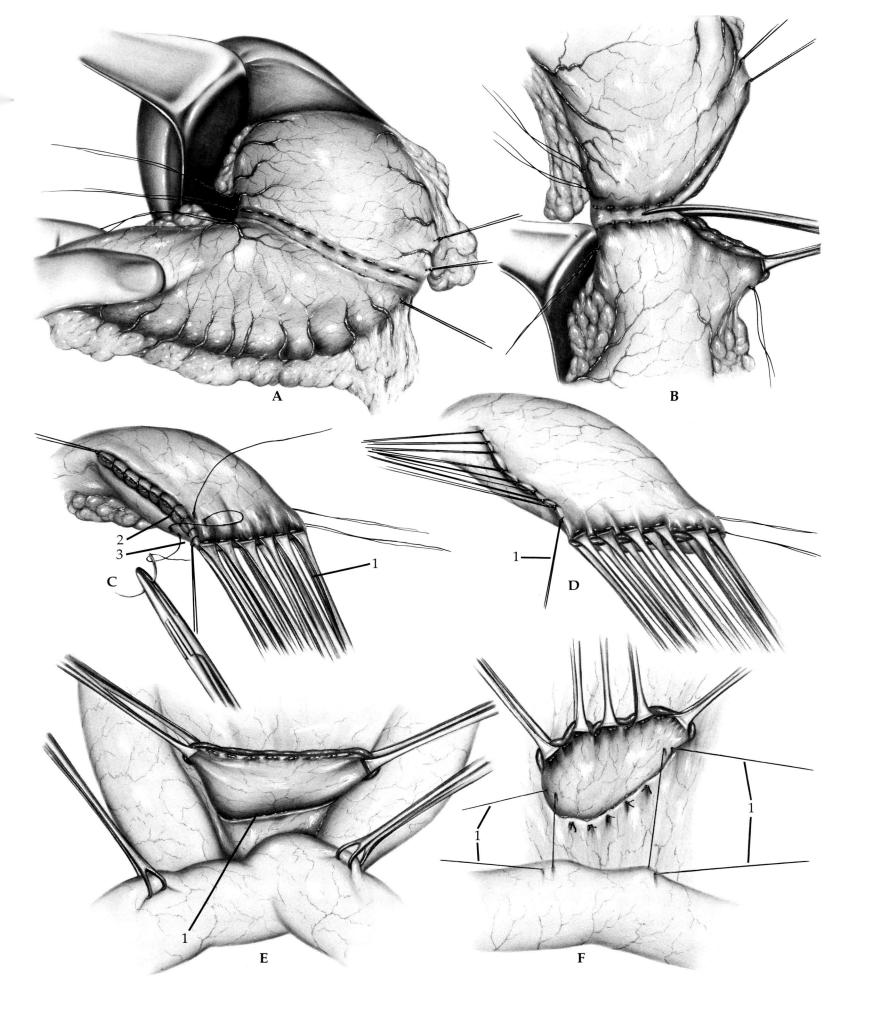

A

B

C

2
3

1

D

1

E

1

F

1

1

PLATE 24 • GASTROJEJUNOSTOMY, BILLROTH II PRINCIPLE, MODIFIED POLYA METHOD—cont'd

Before planning the first anastomotic suture the ligament of Treitz is inspected and is carefully divided to eliminate complicating folds that might serve to angulate the jejunum as it is drawn upward for the anastomosis.

A A 6-inch afferent loop for the anastomosis is approximated to the gastric portion with interrupted Lembert sutures of 3-0 silk.

B The corner stay sutures are used for traction, and the gastric portion is held straight up by the assistant.

C A seromuscular incision across the stomach exposes the gastric intramural vessels, which are clamped with fine Halsted hemostats (1), divided, and tied.

D The gastric mucosa is then opened, and traction is employed on the remaining Allis forceps attached to the line of staples. The corner stay suture (1) from the closure of the lesser curvature and the corner stay suture from the posterior outer row of silk sutures (2) are allowed to remain. A continuous catgut suture is placed along the posterior border of the anastomosis, and is continued anteriorly as an inverting continuous suture after controlling and dividing the gastric vessels in the manner used on the posterior row. Interrupted silks complete the anterior layer.

E With traction on the anastomosis to the right, the "dangerous angle" (1) is exposed. One stay suture from the posterior row (3) and one from the lesser curvature closure (2) identify the area to be reenforced.

F A silk mattress suture is placed through the stomach and jejunum.

G The same suture is continued around the stay sutures, thereby strengthening the angle of the anastomosis.

H The defect in the mesentery is completely closed, and the opening is comfortable. The afferent loop is not twisted, and the suture line is exactly parallel to the mesentric edge of the jejunum.

The duodenal stump is inspected and is reenforced with omental tags, and a drain is placed deep to the duodenal closure.

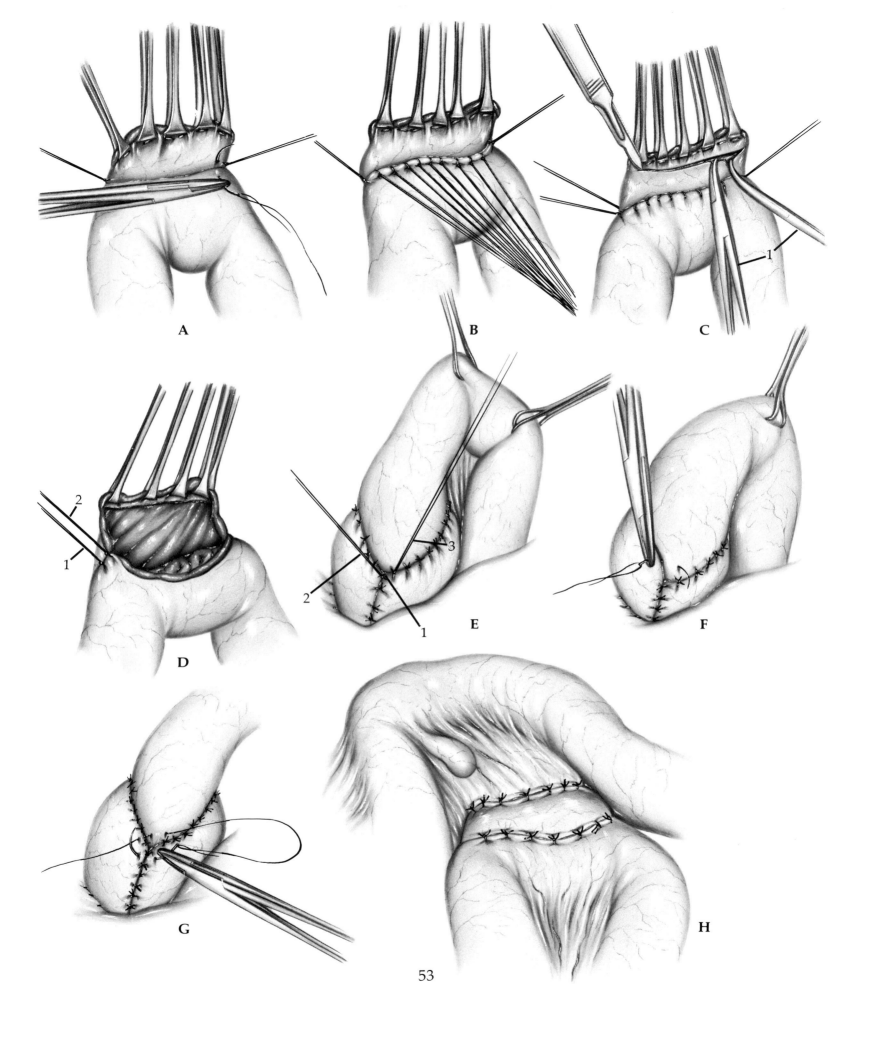

A

B

C

D

E

F

G

H

4

Surgical decompression of the gastric pouch

The use of a temporary gastrostomy for decompression of the intact stomach or gastric remnant after gastric resection is based on sound physiologic grounds. It has been well documented that air swallowing is markedly increased when nasogastric tubes are used. It has been suggested that this increase results from dysfunction of the esophageal constrictors and alterations in the mechanisms of swallowing and respiratory exchange. It has also been shown that nasogastric tube causes increased stimulation of secretions from the mouth and pharynx. In addition esophageal reflux tends to occur when the tube is in place. Use of the gastrostomy tube eliminates the patient discomfort commonly associated with nasogastric suction. Pulmonary toilet in those patients with chronic pulmonary disease such as bronchitis and emphysema is handled with much greater ease in the absence of the nasogastric tube.

PLATE 25 • GASTROSTOMY

A The greater curvature of the stomach is mobilized into the abdominal wound; Babcock clamps are applied, and the mobility of the stomach is determined to be adequate so that the stomach will reach the peritoneum without tension.

B The gastrostomy site is chosen and a purse-string suture *(1)* of 3-0 silk is placed.

C A nephrostomy tube is used for the gastrostomy drainage. This tube is particularly suited for this function because it can be adequately positioned within the stomach for more efficient collection of swallowed air and gastric secretion. A balloon is also present in the system that can be used for additional traction against the abdominal wall. Prior to insertion of the tube, the balloon is carefully tested.

D A stab wound is made in the greater curvature, and the tube is positioned within the stomach.

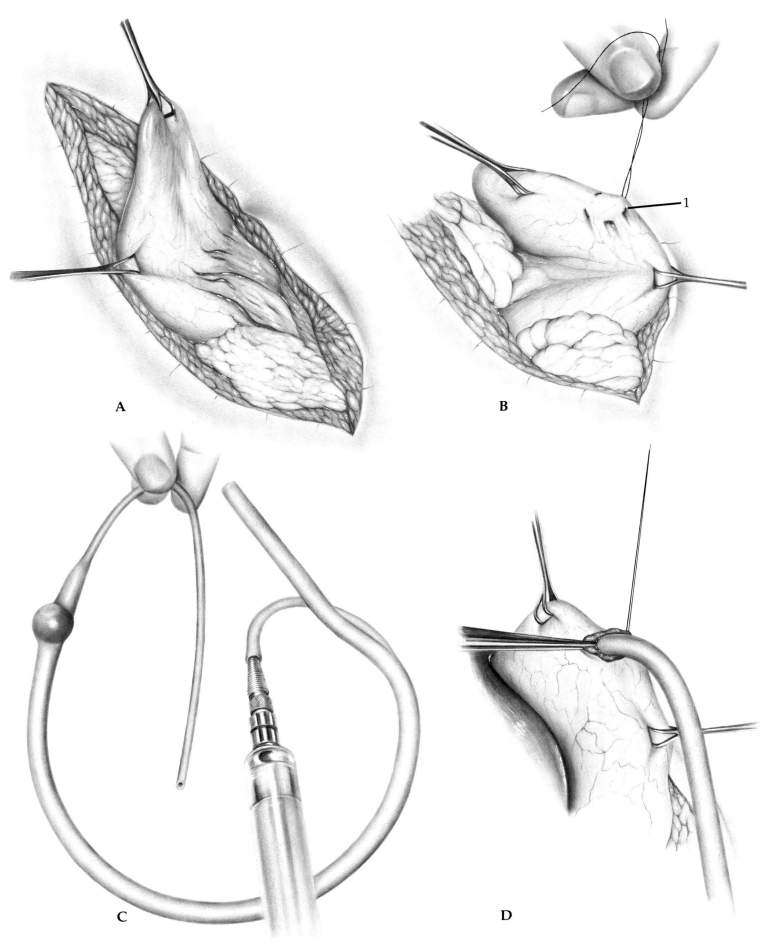

A

B

1

C

D

PLATE 26 • GASTROSTOMY—cont'd

A A second purse-string suture is now being placed.

B The area within the second purse-string suture is slightly inverted, and the suture is tied. This provides an adequate seal for the gastrostomy site.

C The peritoneum and fascial layers are grasped with hemostats and placed on tension.

D A stab wound is made in the abdominal wall with the fascia and peritoneum under tension. The tension serves to maintain proper alignment of the layers of the abdominal wall.

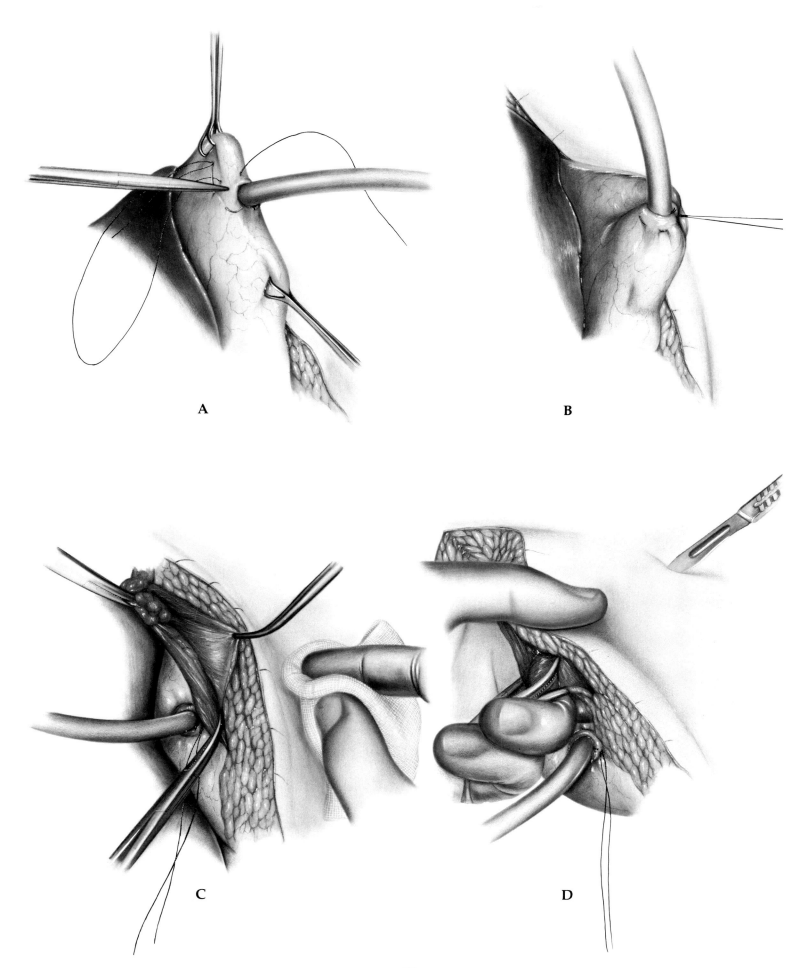

A

B

C

D

59

PLATE 27 • GASTROSTOMY — cont'd

A The gastrostomy tube is drawn through the stab wound in the abdominal wall.

B Interrupted silk sutures *(1)* are used to attach the gastric wall and the parietal peritoneum. Note the persistent traction on the peritoneum and the fascia *(2)*.

C The most lateral sutures securing the stomach have been inserted, tied, and cut. The completion of the attachment of the stomach to the peritoneum is shown here. Note that these sutures are not tied until they have all been inserted.

D With the stomach now securely attached to the posterior aspect of the abdominal wall, the risk of leakage has been eliminated.

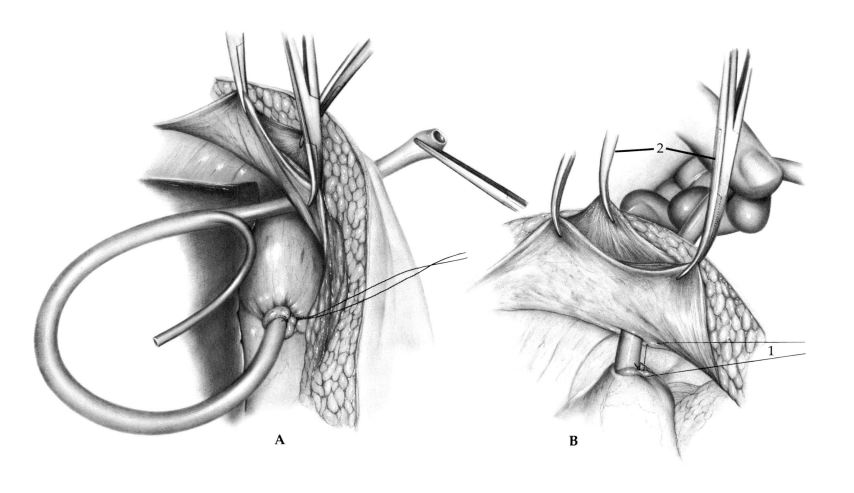

A

B

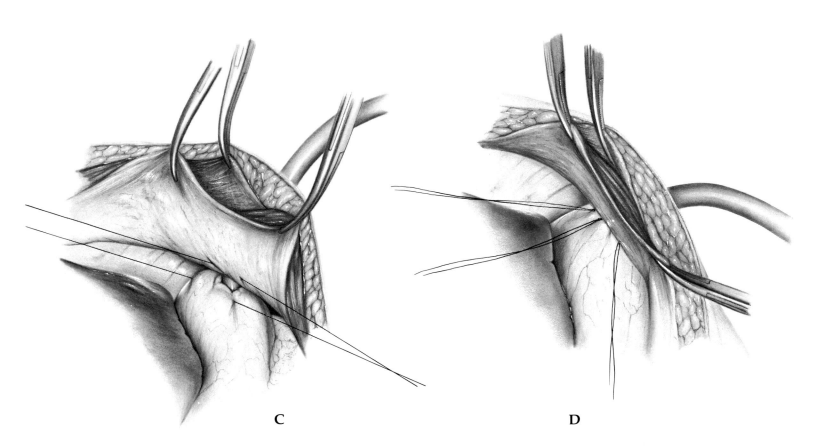

C

D

61

5

Gastric drainage

As an alternative to gastric resection, vagotomy and drainage procedures may be used in patients with peptic ulcer disease. In some centers vagotomy and pyloroplasty or vagotomy and gastroenterostomy is the treatment of choice of most patients with duodenal ulceration. In others this less formidable procedure is reserved for the poor-risk patient, the patient who is thin, or the patient who enters with acute gastrointestinal bleeding. Two criteria must be met for success: first, vagotomy must be complete, thus eliminating the cephalic phase of gastric secretion and, second, a method of gastric drainage that will assure satisfactory gastric emptying and thus prevent antral stasis must be provided. Pyloroplasty has been preferred. Pyloroplasty preserves the normal continuity of the gastrointestinal tract and is also less subject to alkaline reflux into the antrum. When pyloroplasty is not technically feasible, either because of extensive scarring in the area of the duodenum or because of obstruction distal to the point of pyloroplasty, gastroenterostomy provides a generally satisfactory alternative.

PLATE 28 • PYLOROPLASTY

A Kocher maneuver should be done to increase mobility of the duodenum (Plate 9, C). Additional mobility may be gained by release of the lateral attachment of the omentum from the first portion of the duodenum.

A Sutures are placed through the wall of the stomach and duodenum; these sutures serve to mark the extent of incision and to provide a later reference point for the middle of the transverse pyloroplasty closure.

B An incision extending from the gastric suture to the duodenal suture is made; the incision extends for approximately 3.5 cm. on the gastric side and for a slightly shorter distance on the duodenal side. All bleeding points are secured by means of transfixing sutures of 3-0 silk.

C After the intramural vessels have been first clamped and then tied, the mucosa is incised. Babcock clamps are placed at the midpoint of the incision as shown. Traction on these clamps converts the longitudinal defect into a transverse one.

D Inverting Connell sutures of 3-0 silk are placed, and a row of 3-0 silk Lembert sutures reenforces the closure. As an alternative a single layer closure with Weinbergor Gambee sutures may be used.

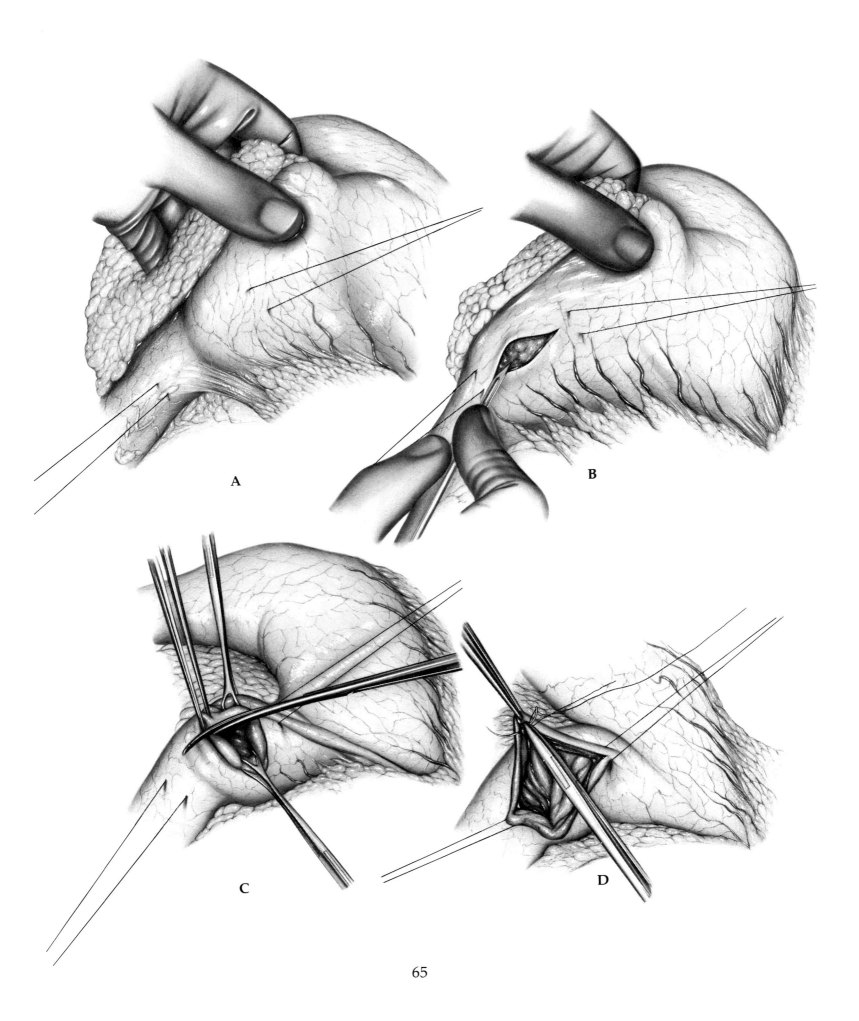

A

B

C

D

PLATE 29 • GASTROJEJUNOSTOMY FOR GASTRIC DRAINAGE

In the event that gastroenterostomy is chosen rather than pyloroplasty for decompressing the vagotomized stomach, several important features of gastroenterostomy will be emphasized in the following description of the operation.

A The surgeon's left hand can be seen here identing the anterior surface of the stomach, with the right index finger pointing at the dependent portion of the stomach where the gastroenterostomy will be performed.

B After the omentum has been separated from the transverse colon as previously described in Plate 6, the posterior aspect of the stomach can now be examined. The examining hand can be seen here with the fingers indenting the gastric wall from the posterior aspect. It is important to perform this maneuver to make certain that there are no overlooked areas of disease in the posterior stomach wall which cannot otherwise be felt adequately.

C After having mobilized the stomach adequately and divided the omentum from the transverse colon, the ligament of Treitz is being shown divided. It is important to divide the ligament of Treitz to avoid angulation of the proximal jejunum and to make it possible to construct a short afferent loop.

D With Babcock clamps placed on the proximal jejunum, the transverse colon is elevated by the hands of the assistant. The loop of proximal jejunum held in the Babcock clamps is shown adjacent to the transverse mesocolon at a site where the stomach will be ultimately brought through the mesocolon to be anastomosed to the jejunum.

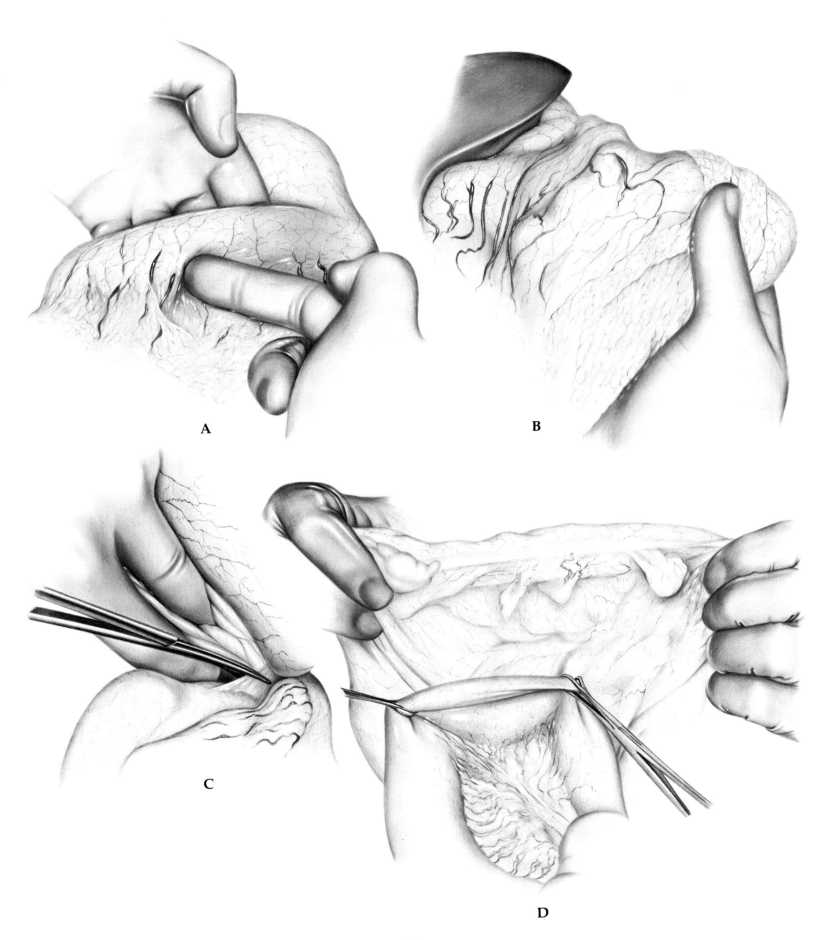

A

B

C

D

67

PLATE 30 • GASTROJEJUNOSTOMY FOR GASTRIC DRAINAGE—cont'd

A An opening has been made in the transverse mesocolon, taking care to avoid the major branches of the middle colic artery; hemostats *(1)* can be seen placed on the small branches of the middle colic artery. By looking through the opening in the transverse mesocolon, the stomach can be seen superior to it.

B The previously described dependent portion of the stomach is grasped with Babcock clamps *(1)*. The stomach is pulled inferiorly through the previously created hole in the mesocolon in preparation for anastomosis to the jejunum, which can be seen below *(2)*.

C The edges of the defect in the mesocolon are now sutured circumferentially to the stomach with interrupted sutures of 3-0 black silk. The first suture is being inserted.

D As the edges of the mesocolic defect are sutured to the stomach, the sutures are shown being placed approximately 1 cm. apart. Care must be taken during the insertion of these sutures not to injure important branches of the middle colic artery.

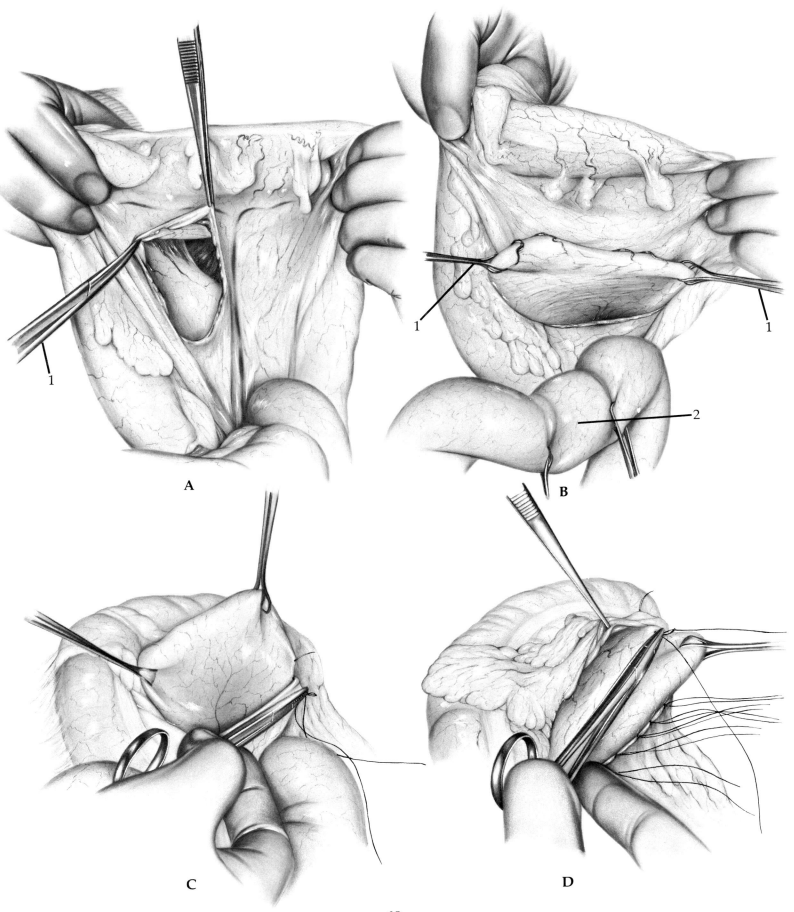

A

B

C

D

69

PLATE 31 • GASTROJEJUNOSTOMY FOR GASTRIC DRAINAGE—cont'd

A After the stomach has been securely fixed to the edges of the opening in the mesocolon, the gastrojejunostomy is continued. Noncrushing intestinal clamps *(1)* are placed across a portion of the stomach and of the jejunum to prevent spillage of gastrointestinal contents and to control hemorrhage during the course of the anastomosis. As the gastroenterostomy is begun, a black silk suture *(2)* can be seen being inserted in a horizontal mattress fashion through the jejunum.

B The first seromuscular suture has been completed and can now be seen inserted in both the jejunum and the stomach. These sutures are tied as they are placed.

C The entire row of seromuscular sutures has now been inserted and tied, and the length of the gastrojejunostomy has been outlined by the two corner sutures *(1)*.

D With the gastrointestinal clamps still in place, an incision is made in the jejunum parallel to the previously inserted line of seromuscular sutures. A scalpel is chosen for making this incision, and the glass suction tip *(1)* can be seen to aspirate the small amount of bleeding that will be encountered as the incision progresses.

E After having incised the seromuscular layer of the intestine and stomach, the mucosa is grasped with the forceps *(1)*, and the incision into the lumen of the bowel is completed with the scissors. The same maneuver is carried out on the gastric side.

F The jejunum and the stomach have now been opened for similar lengths. Note that the seromuscular sutures are still intact and are used for traction in preparation for completing the portion of the anastomosis approximating the mucus membrane. Babcock clamps *(1)* are placed on the edge of the jejunum and stomach to facilitate completion of the anastomosis.

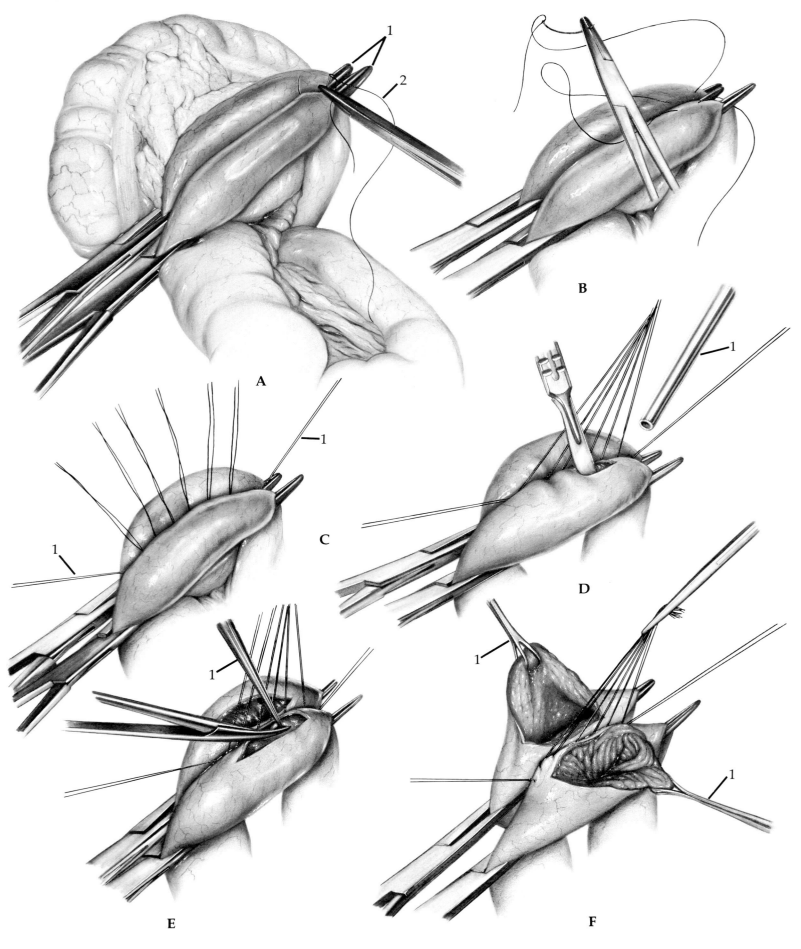

A

B

C

D

E

F

PLATE 32 • GASTROJEJUNOSTOMY FOR GASTRIC DRAINAGE—cont'd

A The inner layer of the posterior part of the anastomosis is now begun, starting in the corner of the anastomosis most distal from the surgeon. A 3-0 or 4-0 silk suture is inserted through the full thickness of the jejunum and the full thickness of the stomach. Note again the exposure accomplished by the Babcock clamps placed on the cut edge of the jejunum and stomach.

B After the first mucosa-approximating suture has been inserted, the previously tied seromuscular sutures are divided in turn.

C As the posterior part of the anastomosis is completed, the mucosa-approximating sutures can be seen being inserted through the full thickness of the wall of the stomach and the jejunum.

D Again note that the previously placed seromuscular sutures are cut in order as the mucosa-approximating suture line is continued.

E The posterior part of the anastomosis is now completed, and the sutures approximating the mucosa can be seen being held in a clamp.

F The mucosa-approximating sutures have now been divided, and the surgeon is ready to begin the anterior portion of the anastomosis.

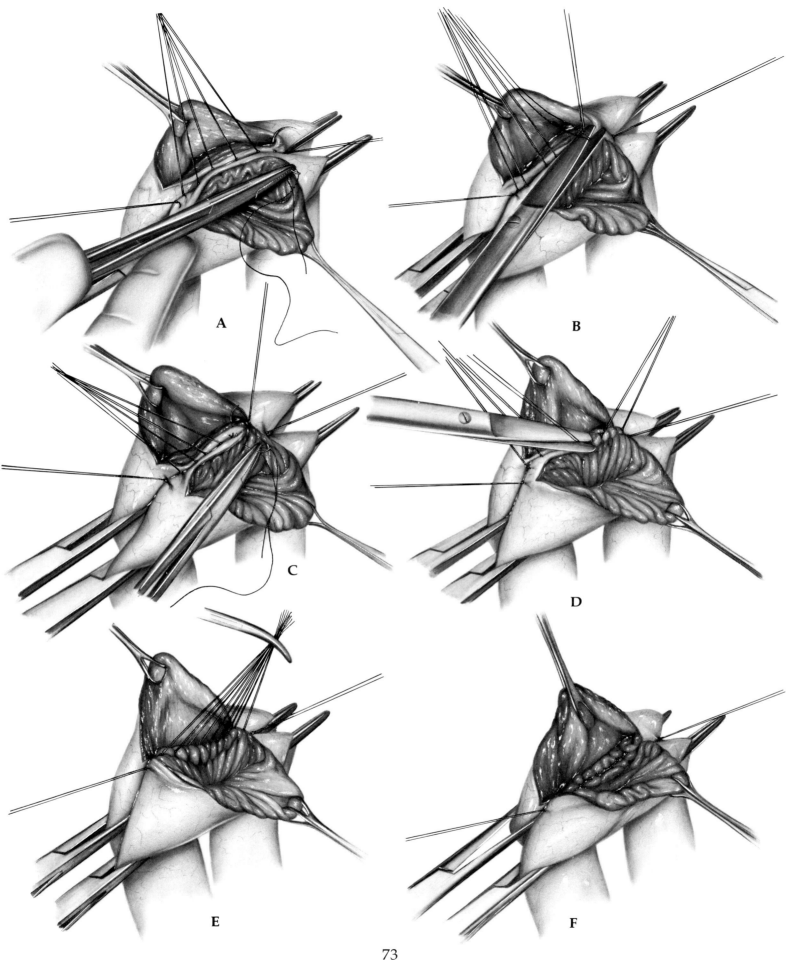

A

B

C

D

E

F

73

PLATE 33 • GASTROJEJUNOSTOMY FOR GASTRIC DRAINAGE—cont'd

The method of inverting the gastrojejunostomy is identical to that described in Plates 19 and 20 dealing with gastroduodenostomy. The reader is referred to those Plates for the details of the completion of the anastomosis.

A After the inversion of the anterior portion of the anastomosis has been completed, reinforcement is accomplished by a row of Lembert sutures. Note that the intestinal clamps have been removed from the stomach and jejunum, since there is no longer any danger of spillage.

B The anterior portion of the anastomosis is now completed, and the row of Lembert sutures can be seen tied but not yet cut.

C Attention is now directed to the corners of the anastomosis, and a reinforcing suture is inserted.

D The technique for reinforcing the corner is clearly shown here, and the reinforcing suture has been placed but not tied until the previous corner stitch (1) is divided. The other corner of the anastomosis is handled in a similar fashion.

E After reinforcements of the corners have been completed, the surgeon inspects the anastomosis manually to make certain that it is patent.

F The gastrojejunostomy having been completed, the anastomotic line can be seen with the opening in the mesocolon sutured to the stomach proximal to it.

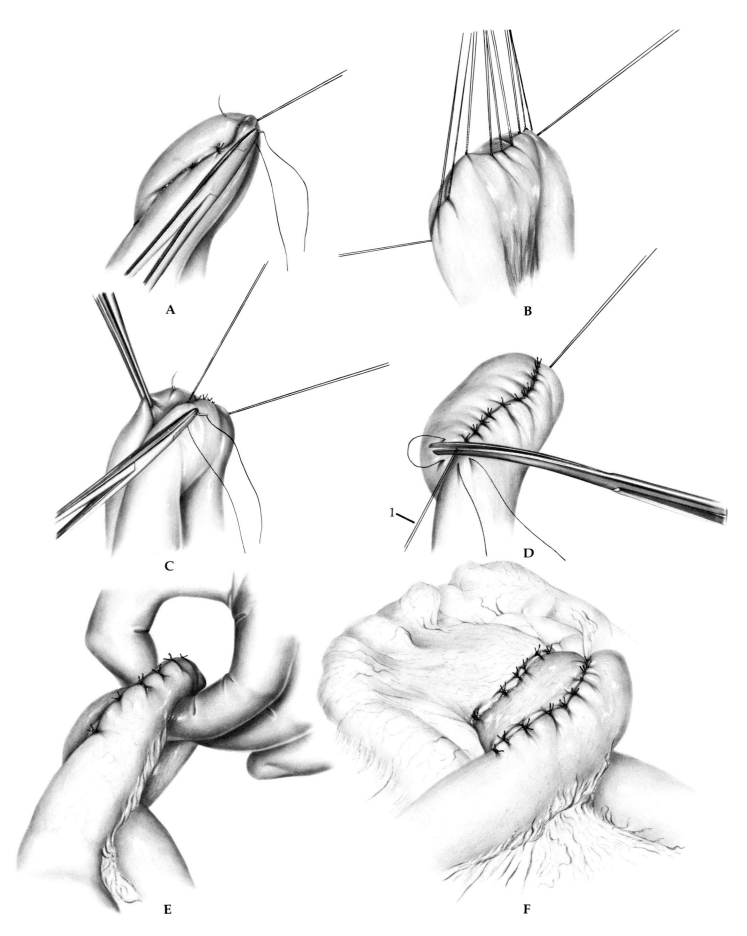

A

B

C

D

1

E

F

75

CHAPTER
6

Gastrotomy

A mass in the stomach requires definitive diagnosis before intelligent decisions can be made concerning surgical therapy. The following is a description of a method for biopsying intragastric lesions.

PLATE 34 • GASTROTOMY

A The mass is identified by palpation, and the extent of gastric involvement is determined. It is important to perform a bimanual examination of all gastric masses, and the examination of the posterior aspect of the stomach is particularly important (Plate 29). In this demonstration the intragastric mass can be seen outlined by the surgeon's examining hand in the midportion of the stomach.

B The incision is begun in the stomach with the scalpel, as demonstrated in Plate 31, D. After the gastric mucosa has been identified, the remainder of the gastrotomy is performed with the scissors. Babcock clamps *(1)* are then used to grasp the cut edges of the stomach. It is preferable to make the gastrotomy in the long axis of the stomach so that it may be extended as required. Occasionally a transverse gastrotomy is permissible if the extent of the lesion is quite clear prior to opening the stomach.

C After the stomach has been opened, the surgeon's left index finger is used to stabilize the intragastric lesion while a scalpel performs an incisional biopsy. Note that the tumor mass is not grasped with an instrument to avoid distortion of the histology of the lesion in question.

D After the specimen has been biopsied and the diagnosis confirmed with a frozen section, the incision in the stomach is closed with interrupted through-and-through black silk sutures.

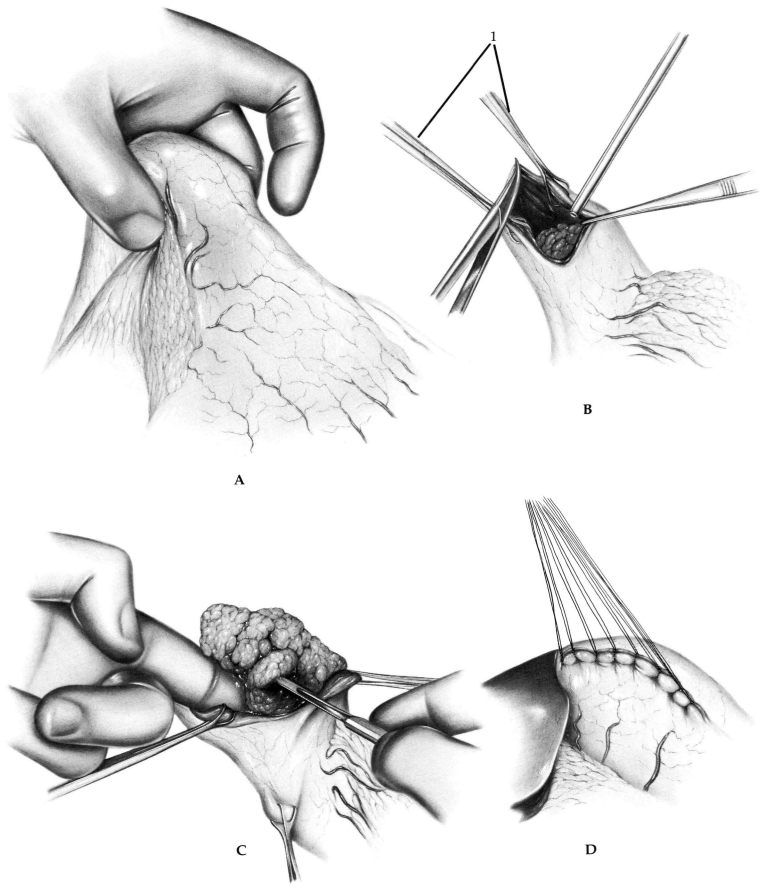

CHAPTER

7

Wedge resection

Surgical therapy for a benign gastric ulcer located high on the lesser curvature or near the gastroesophageal junction will usually require an extensive gastric resection. In a poor-risk patient, particularly one who is thin, a wedge resection of the ulcer may be applicable. A subdiaphragmatic vagotomy is first done not only to decrease parietal cell sensitivity and to block gastrin release, but also for mobilization and exposure of the upper portion of the stomach. When a vagotomy is done, a drainage procedure (pyloroplasty) must also be performed in conjunction.

PLATE 35 • WEDGE RESECTION

A The position of the patient and the incision are the same as shown for vagotomy and subtotal resection (Plates 1 to 4). The surgeon must first ascertain the feasibility of a wedge resection. This procedure is not indicated in carcinoma of the stomach. The surgeon is shown palpating the area of the ulcer high on the lesser curvature of the stomach.

B Since in most cases the indication for wedge resection is a very high, lesser curvature gastric ulcer, the area should first be well exposed. A broad retractor is placed just to the left of the xiphoid with upward and outward retraction applied under the left costal margin. A second broad retractor or Deaver retractor is placed to the right and retracts the left lobe of the liver. A bilateral subdiaphragmatic truncal vagotomy is necessary to provide mobilization of the esophagocardial junction. The area of the abdominal esophagus is exposed as in Plates 2 to 4. The anterior trunk is shown divided between two long right-angle clamps placed 1 to 2 cm. apart. A forceps (1) grasps the section of vagus nerve that is to be removed. Histologic evidence of two nerve trunks does not ensure that a complete vagotomy has been performed, since there are frequently accessory trunks.

C A 2-0 silk suture ligature may be used to transfix the ends of the nerve trunks. Often small vessels accompany these trunks, and this prevents troublesome bleeding.

D In addition to vagotomy, division of the gastrohepatic ligament is a necessary step to completely mobilize the uppermost portion of the lesser curvature. Division of the gastrohepatic ligament (1) is made between two clamps. Small branches of the left gastric artery pass through the gastrohepatic ligament to supply the abdominal portion of the esophagus, so ligation of the divided ends is required.

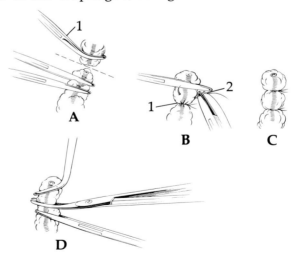

A, The technique shown here is used for the safe handling of potentially dangerous vessels. Three clamps are used, with one being a right angle (1). **B,** A ligature is tied (1) followed by a distal suture ligature (2). **C,** The completed process is shown. **D,** The ease of dividing between clamps, when clamps with different curves are used, is shown.

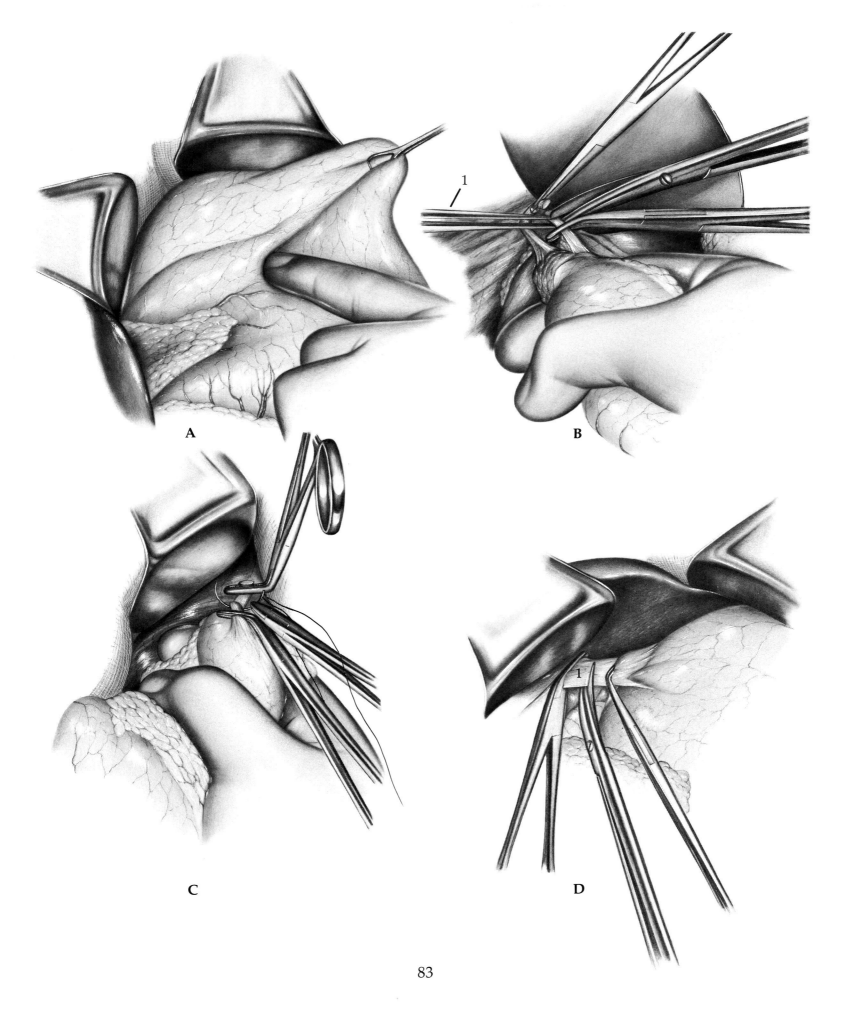

A

B

1

C

D

1

1

83

PLATE 36 • WEDGE RESECTION — cont'd

A A Babcock clamp *(1)* grasps the anterior wall of the stomach body to provide some traction of the gastrosplenic mesentery. A forceps *(2)* is shown elevating an avascular segment of the gastrosplenic mesentery, through which an opening is made with a Metzenbaum scissors *(3)*.

B The opening into the lesser sac is extended by dividing segments of the gastrosplenic mesentery between clamps. This mesentery is manipulated with care, since it attaches to the splenic capsule, and excessive traction may result in a tear of the capsule and in troublesome bleeding.

C The divided ends are ligated with 2-0 silk transfixing sutures. The opening should be extended to admit the surgeon's hand and retractors if necessary.

D Entry into the lesser sac provides exposure to the posterior wall of the stomach *(1)*, the posterior lesser curvature area, and the pancreas *(2)*. The surgeon is shown palpating the body of the pancreas.

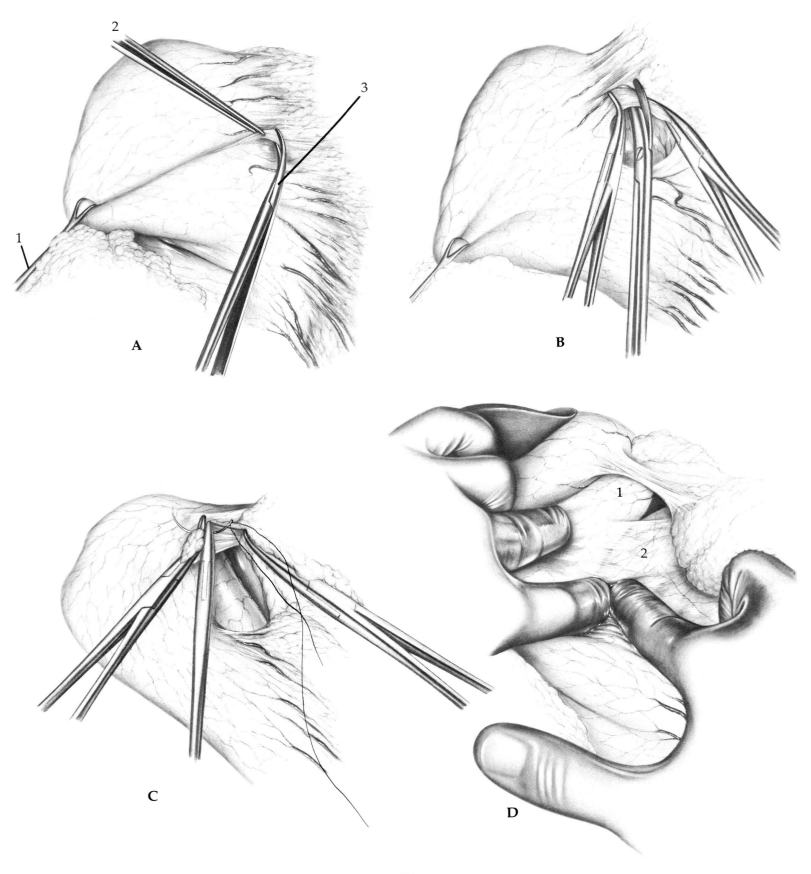

A

B

C

D

85

PLATE 37 • WEDGE RESECTION—cont'd

A Further exposure of the lesser curvature area on the underside of the stomach is obtained by division of the thin avascular peritoneal folds that usually are present and attach the posterior stomach *(1)* to the capsule of the underlying pancreas *(2)*.

B These attachments are thin and veillike and can be quickly divided with scissors dissection.

C The surgeon's hand shown placed under the stomach can palpate the entire posterior aspect of the stomach and lesser curvature. The fingertip is shown as it is passed through an avascular area of the lesser omentum away from the lesser curvature.

D Through the opening in the lesser omentum, the surgeon's left hand, with the index finger posterior and thumb on the anterior aspect of the lesser curvature, bimanually palpates the ulcer area along the lesser curvature.

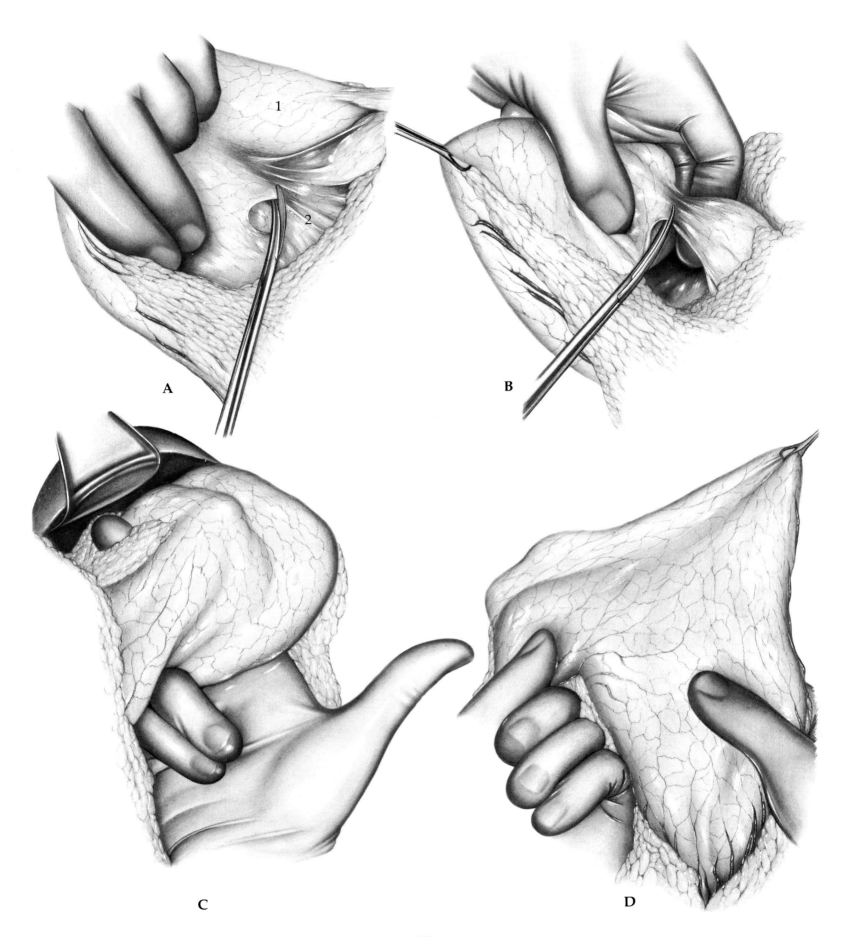

A

B

C

D

87

PLATE 38 • WEDGE RESECTION—cont'd

A The surgeon's fingertip guides a Kelly clamp *(1)* under the left gastric vessels high on the lesser curvature and 2 to 5 cm. above the area to be excised. The dotted lines indicate the area to be wedged out.

B The left gastric vessels and lesser omentum are divided between clamps. These vessels are ligated with 2-0 silk transfixing sutures. A double clamp technique may be used (illustrated on page 82).

C Several centimeters below the ulcer area along the lesser curvature the right gastric artery and adjacent lesser omentum are similarly dissected free and divided between clamps.

D Transfixing sutures of 2-0 silk are placed to ligate the divided ends of the right gastric vessels. An area through the lesser omentum and the vessels along the lesser curvature have been divided both above and below the segment of lesser curvature that will be excised in a wedge fashion.

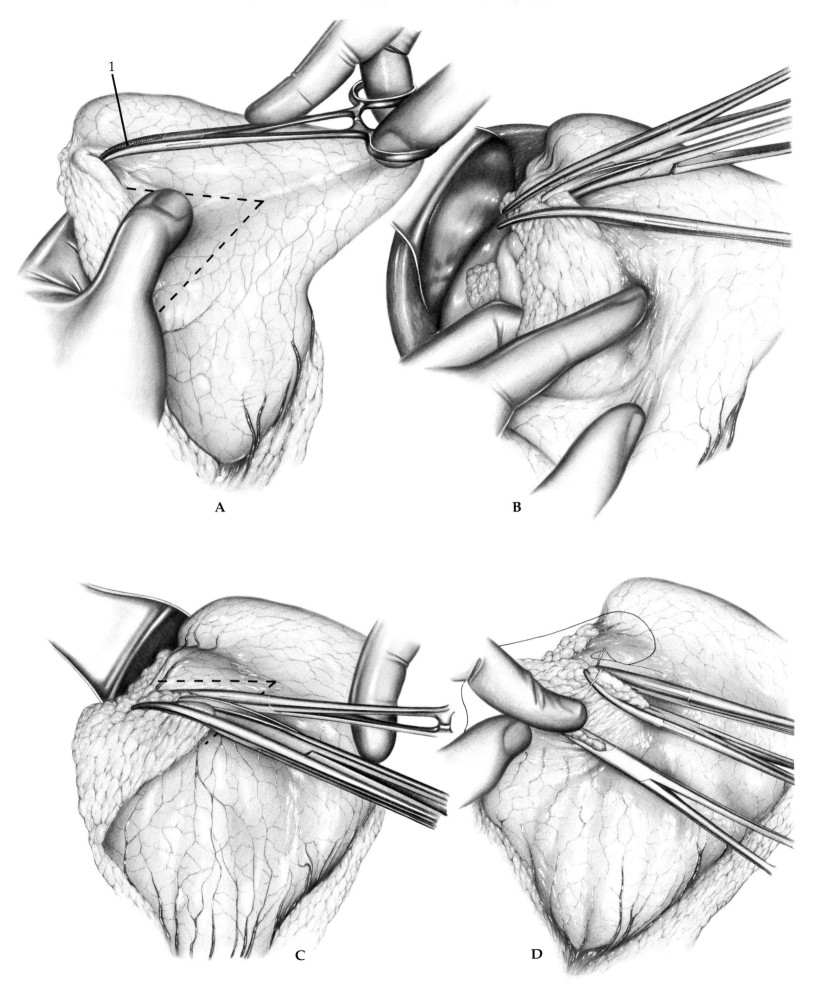

A

B

C

D

89

PLATE 39 • WEDGE RESECTION — cont'd

A The lesser curvature has been mobilized, and the lesser omentum has been divided above and below the area of planned resection. A 2-0 silk suture is placed through the full thickness of the anterior stomach wall 5 to 6 cm. away from the ulcer area, indicated in *A* to *C* by the ×. This suture marks the apex of the wedge resection. A Babcock clamp *(1)* elevates the anterior wall to facilitate placement of the sutures. The surgeon should avoid picking up the posterior stomach wall with these sutures.

B The line of sutures is continued medially, crossing above the ulcer to the lesser curvature near the point of the previously divided left gastric vessels and lesser omentum. The suture ends of this row are tagged with a small hemostat.

C A second row of sutures is placed below the ulcer. These sutures form a triangle, with the base of the triangle along the lesser curvature and the apex pointing toward the greater curvature. The area with the ulcer is encompassed by the sutures. A small hemostat *(1)* tags the suture ends.

D The Babcock clamp *(1)* is shown grasping the margin of the greater curvature. The greater curvature *(2)* has been lifted upward, exposing the posterior wall of the stomach *(3)*. Two rows of 2-0 silk sutures are similarly placed through the posterior wall of the stomach around the ulcer area *(4)*. The wedge of stomach to be removed has now been completely outlined by sutures placed in both the anterior and posterior gastric wall.

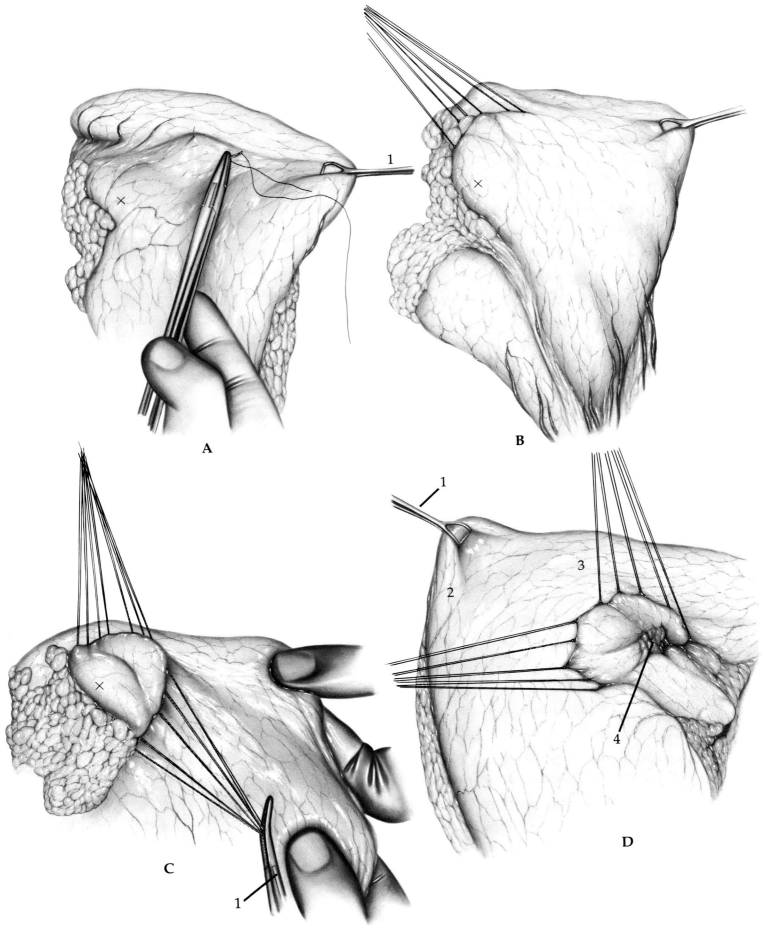

A

B

C

1

1

D

1

2

3

4

91

PLATE 40 • WEDGE RESECTION—cont'd

A The lesser curvature area to be excised is surrounded by the through-and-through sutures. The two rows in the anterior wall of the stomach are shown. These sutures will provide both hemostasis and traction. The stomach is opened with scissors *(1)*, starting below the ulcer, but above the distal row of sutures.

B The entire area encompassed by the anterior wall sutures is opened. The ulcer *(1)* along the lesser curvature can be seen. A suture *(2)* has been placed through the apex of the anterior wall for traction.

C The tagged ends of the posterior wall sutures *(1)* are passed under the stomach and up through the opening along the lesser curvature in the lesser omentum. Traction on the tagged ends of the posterior two rows of sutures elevates the lesser curvature area with the ulcer *(2)*. The posterior wall area encompassed by sutures and the lesser curvature can now be excised with good visualization of the margins. A four-quadrant area biopsy of the ulcer should be performed. Before closing the defect, the nasogastric tube *(3)* is repositioned. The ends of the hemostatic sutures are cut.

D The defect created by the wedge resection is closed in two layers, using interrupted 2-0 silk sutures. The first row sutures are placed through all layers of both edges of the opening. The final outside row of 2-0 silk Lembert sutures is illustrated.

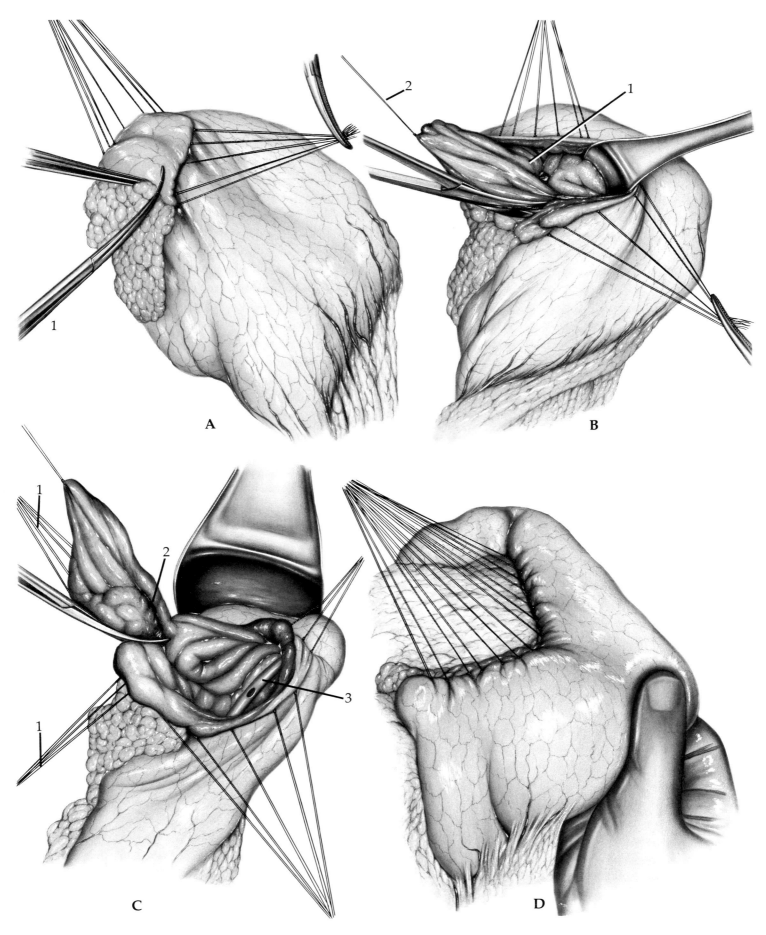

CHAPTER
8

Total gastrectomy

Total gastrectomy may be indicated in malignancies of the proximal stomach or when the tumor involves most of the lesser curvature. When total gastrectomy is applied for malignant lesions, the entire stomach, the first part of the duodenum, the greater and lesser omentum, the spleen and often the distal pancreas, and a portion of distal esophagus are resected en bloc. When total gastrectomy is performed to remove the target organ of a gastrin-producing islet cell tumor (Zollinger-Ellison syndrome), as these plates illustrate, then the resection need not be as radical. The position of the patient, incision, and initial mobilization of the stomach are as shown in Plates 2 to 9.

PLATE 41 • TOTAL GASTRECTOMY

A The attachment of the greater omentum to the antral area has been dissected free and is now divided between Kelly clamps (Plate 10, *A*).

B While an assistant holds the stomach and greater omentum upward, the surgeon may palpate and dissect free the right gastroepiploic vessels from the distal stomach and duodenum. Previously divided and ligated vessels are shown *(1)*. In addition the small vascular attachments between the duodenum and pancreas are dissected free, divided, and ligated.

C While palpating the right gastric artery with the left hand, the fingertip guides the right-angle clamp beneath the vessels.

D The vessel is divided between clamps, and the vessel ends are ligated with 2-0 silk transfixing sutures.

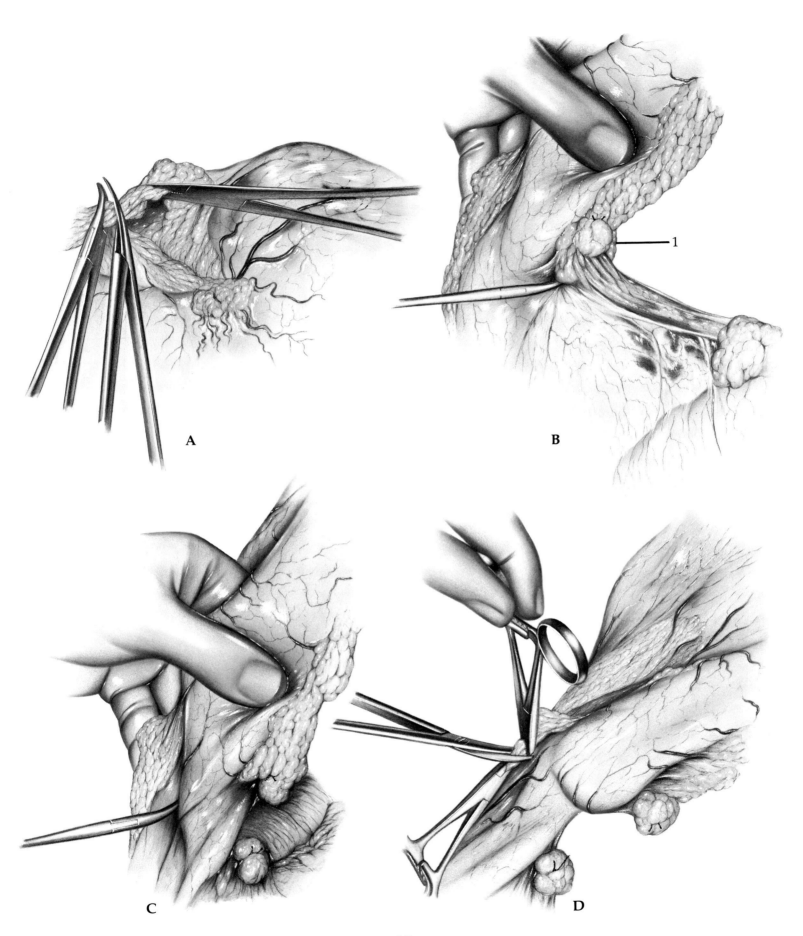

A

B

1

C

D

97

PLATE 42 • TOTAL GASTRECTOMY—cont'd

A A Potts or Glassman noncrushing clamp *(1)* is placed across the duodenum 1 to 2 cm. distal to the pylorus. An additional 2 cm. of duodenum has been cleared distal to the clamp to facilitate closure of the duodenal stump. When carcinoma of the distal stomach is the indication for surgery, then 4 to 6 cm. of the duodenum distal to the pylorus should be included in the resection.

B A Kocher clamp *(1)* is placed across the duodenum proximal to the noncrushing clamp. The duodenum is then divided with a scalpel, leaving a small cuff to prevent the end of the duodenum from slipping through the noncrushing clamp. The suction tip *(2)* aspirates any spillage.

C After dividing the duodenum the divided end of the stomach is lifted upward, exposing the pedicle containing the left gastric artery and vein. This pedicle is doubly clamped prior to division. When gastric carcinoma is the indication for total gastrectomy, then the left gastric artery is divided close to the celiac axis, and the node-bearing tissue is removed en bloc. An 0 silk suture is tied around the pedicle beneath the bottom clamp. The bottom clamp is then removed before removal of the top clamp and a second 2-0 silk transfixing suture is placed distal to the first tie on the divided pedicle. (See page 82.)

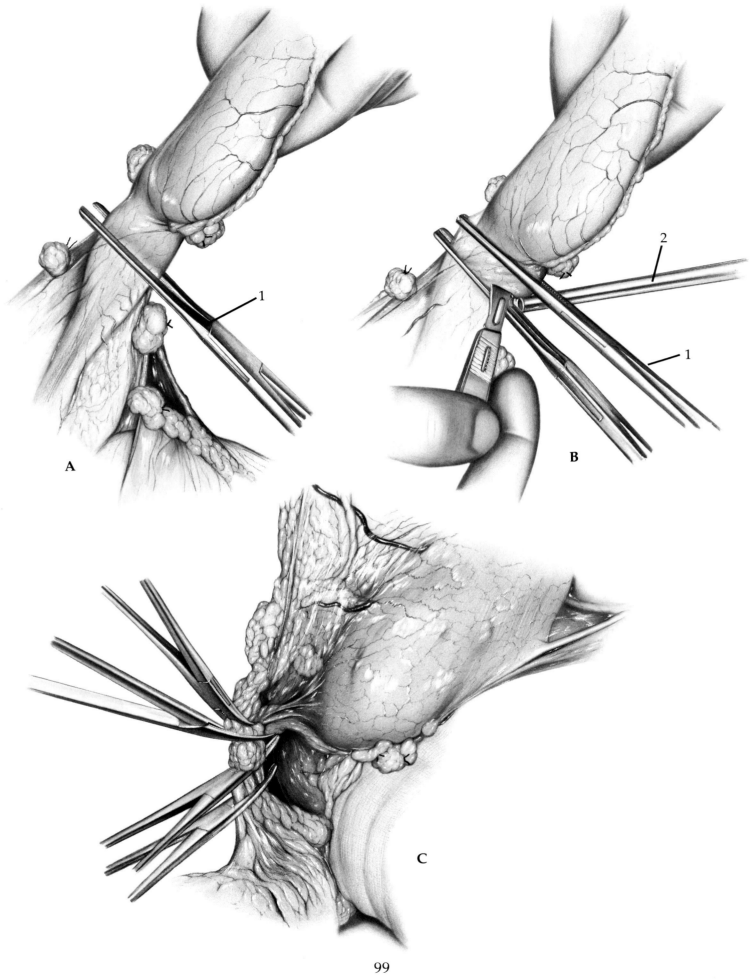

A

B

1

2

1

C

99

PLATE 43 • TOTAL GASTRECTOMY — cont'd

A Prior to closure of the duodenal stump, stay sutures are placed through the corners below the noncrushing clamp.

B Noninverting mattress sutures of 2-0 silk are placed through the end of the divided duodenum below the noncrushing clamp. (An alternative method utilizes interrupted inverting sutures for the first layer.)

C The noncrushing clamp is removed. The ends of the first row of sutures are then cut. The corner sutures are left in place to provide traction facilitating placement of the second row of sutures.

D A second layer of 2-0 silk Lembert sutures is placed to start inverting the first layer closure.

E The needle should bite an adequate amount of the seromuscular layer. Small bites with fine sutures have a tendency to cut through.

F The stump closure has been completed. Note that no excess duodenum has been mobilized.

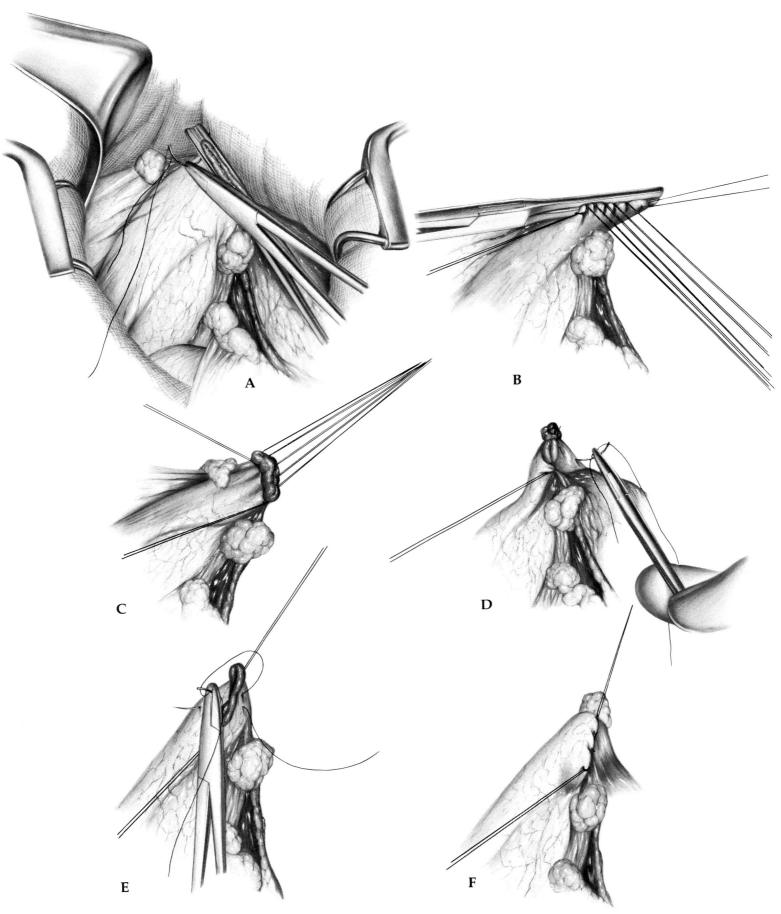

A

B

C

D

E

F

101

PLATE 44 • TOTAL GASTRECTOMY — cont'd

Prior to mobilization of the spleen a ligature is placed around the splenic artery as it passes along the superior border of the tail of the pancreas. This maneuver diminishes the possibility of troublesome bleeding from adhesions to the splenic capsule when removing the spleen from the splenic fossa. Ligation of the splenic artery (but not the splenic vein) at this point in the operation will also allow some of the blood held in the spleen to pass into the patient. The spleen becomes smaller and the patient receives the additional blood, a type of autotransfusion. Exposure to this splenic artery is through the avascular attachment of the omentum on the transverse colon (Plate 6).

A Lateral to this avascular attachment, the gastrocolic ligament and omentum are fused. These are divided between Kelly clamps, and 2-0 silk ligatures transfix the divided ends. Note that one of the clamps is a right angle *(1)* and one is a Kelly *(2)*, facilitating division with the scissors.

B A Deaver retractor is placed over a lap pad on the colon inferiorly, and the stomach is retracted medially.

C The splenic artery courses serpiginously along the superior edge of the pancreas, and its pulsations make it easily palpable. The peritoneum over the splenic artery is elevated with forceps and incised.

D A right-angle clamp is used to bluntly dissect around the artery. A 2-0 silk suture is passed around the splenic artery and tied. The splenic artery is not divided at this point. Although the artery is shown being doubly ligated, a single tie will suffice.

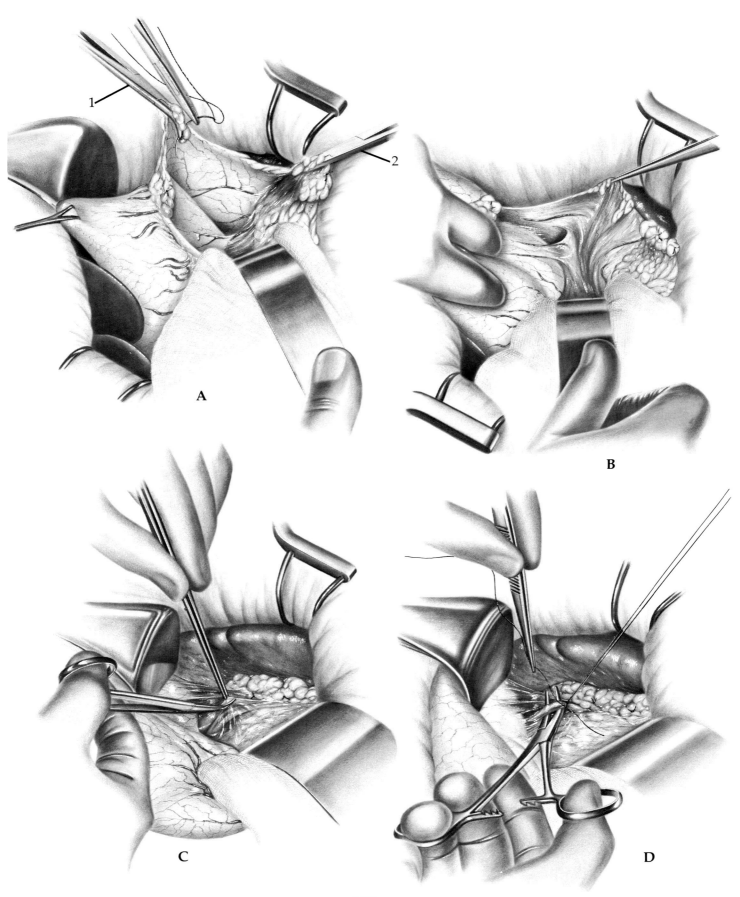

PLATE 45 • TOTAL GASTRECTOMY—cont'd

After division of the splenocolic and lienorenal ligaments and any adhesions (Plate 61), the spleen is delivered from its fossa.

A The spleen is shown still attached to the stomach by the gastrosplenic mesentery so that it may be removed en bloc with the stomach specimen.

B The splenic vessels are divided between Kelly clamps. The tail of the pancreas should be visualized before placement of these or any clamps to avoid injury to pancreatic tissue.

C Several segments will need to be individually clamped and divided.

D Transfixing sutures of 2-0 silk are placed around the divided vessel ends near the tail of the pancreas.

The lymphatics of the greater curvature, fundus, and upper portion of the stomach body drain into lymph nodes at the splenic hilum and along the vessels bordering the tail of the pancreas. If these nodes are obviously involved, the tail of the pancreas should be resected and removed en bloc with the spleen.

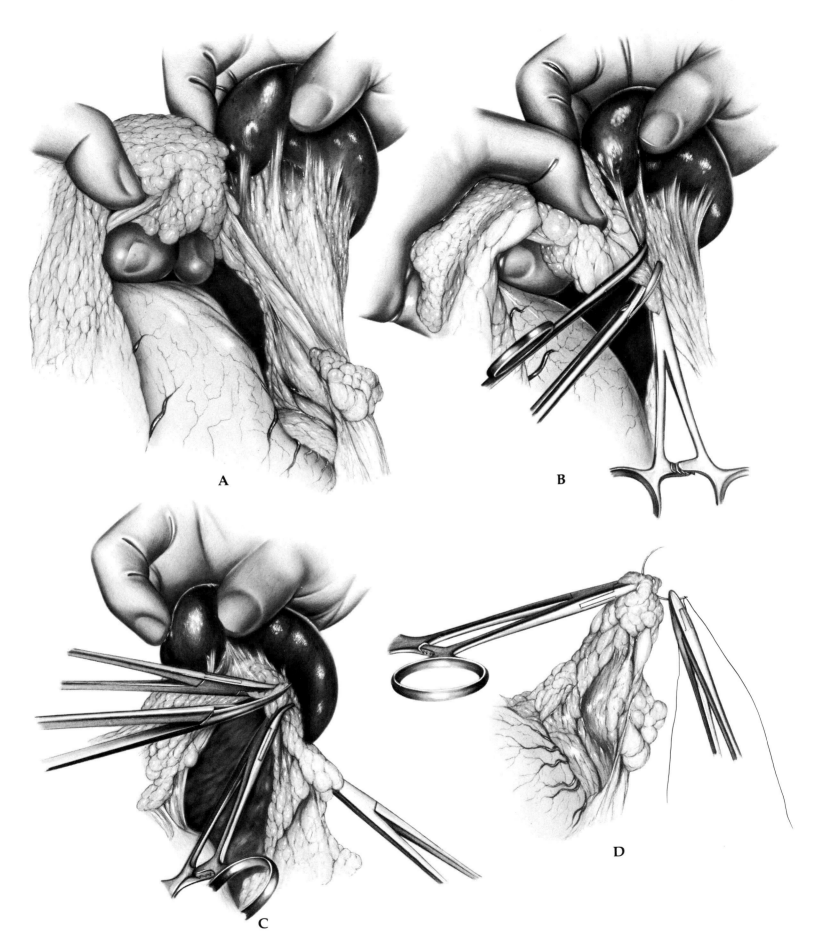

PLATE 46 • TOTAL GASTRECTOMY — cont'd

A An alternative approach at this point is to first remove the spleen without the en bloc technique. When total gastrectomy is done for a gastrin-producing islet cell tumor (Zollinger-Ellison syndrome), an en bloc removal of the spleen and stomach is not usually necessary. The indication for total gastrectomy in the Zollinger-Ellison syndrome is removal of the target organ for gastrin. In this syndrome rarely does the surgeon find a single primary tumor that can be totally excised so that the entire stomach must be removed to control the ulcer diathesis. Mobilization of the spleen is as shown in Plates 60 and 61. Ligation of the splenic artery prior to mobilization of the spleen may diminish any bleeding incurred (Plate 44, *D*). The distal end of pancreas is carefully visualized, and the splenic vessels *(1)* are isolated prior to division of the splenic pedicle.

B The duodenojejunal flexure at the ligament of Treitz is illustrated. The transverse colon and mesocolon have been lifted upward, showing the ascending limb (fourth part) of duodenum and first portion of jejunum. An avascular fold is often present, attaching the top of the duodenojejunal flexure to the base of the mesocolon. This fold is divided with scissors, carefully avoiding injury to the vessels in the mesocolon immediately posterior.

C The first part of the jejunum is held up and folded to the patient's right side, exposing the superior duodenal fold at the junction of the ascending (fourth part) duodenum and jejunum. Division of this avascular fold with Metzenbaum scissors is shown. This completes the additional mobilization of the duodenojejunal flexure, which avoids kinking and potential obstruction in this area when bringing up the afferent limb of jejunum to the esophagus.

D The phrenocolic ligament is divided, which allows mobilization of the splenic flexure of the colon.

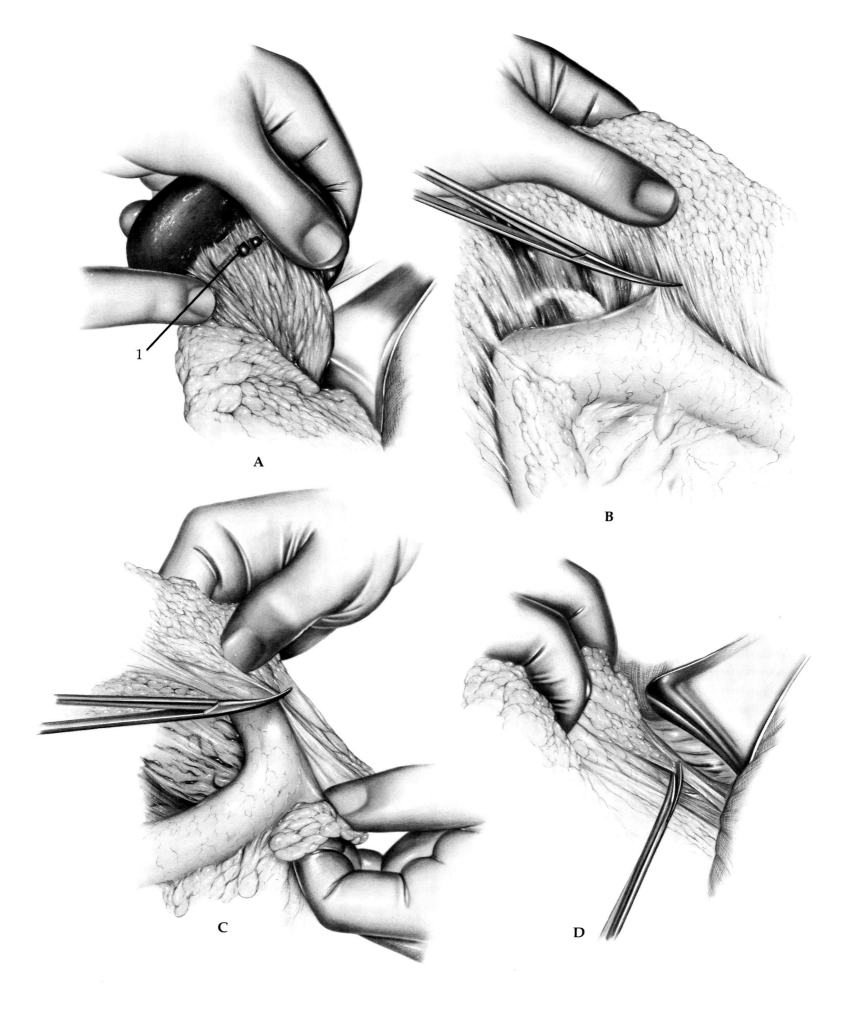

A

B

C

D

PLATE 47 • TOTAL GASTRECTOMY — cont'd

A While the first assistant elevates the transverse colon, the surgeon makes an opening at the base of the transverse mesocolon to the left of the middle colic vessels. Babcock clamps are placed on the antimesenteric border of the jejunum. Placement of these clamps marks the top of the jejunal loop and should allow approximation of the top of the jejunal loop to the esophagus without any tension. The length of the afferent limb varies with the size of the patient. The arrows show the direction of flow of gastrointestinal contents through the jejunum.

B The loop of proximal jejunum is brought through the mesentery, and the stomach is elevated upward, showing the posterior wall of the esophagus. The surgeon then adjusts this loop to allow approximation of its uppermost portion to the esophagus without tension of the afferent limb. Previous mobilization at the duodenojejunal flexure avoids kinking and potential obstruction at the ligament of Treitz (Plate 29, C). Note again the amount of esophagus that has been mobilized into the abdominal cavity. When carcinoma evolves in the proximal stomach or cardiac area, an additional length of esophagus is mobilized down below the diaphragm to avoid construction of the anastomosis in an area of esophagus in which there is intramural spread of tumor.

C Sutures of 2-0 silk on French-eye needles are placed through the seromuscular layer of the antimesenteric border of jejunum. The surgeon should start the posterior row of mattress sutures 1 cm. on the back side of the loop of jejunum so that the opening will be exactly antimesenteric. There is a tendency to place the anastomotic opening too far anterior if the first sutures are placed on the antimesenteric border.

D The suture is then placed horizontally through the full thickness of the esophagus without penetrating the mucosa. The posterior wall of the esophagus and the top of the jejunal loop should approximate without tension. The sutures are not tied down at this point. The ends of each suture are clamped with a small hemostat to keep the sutures neatly separated.

E The row of mattress sutures is continued, suturing toward the surgeon. This row of interrupted sutures will constitute the posterior outer layer of sutures of the esophagojejunal anastomosis.

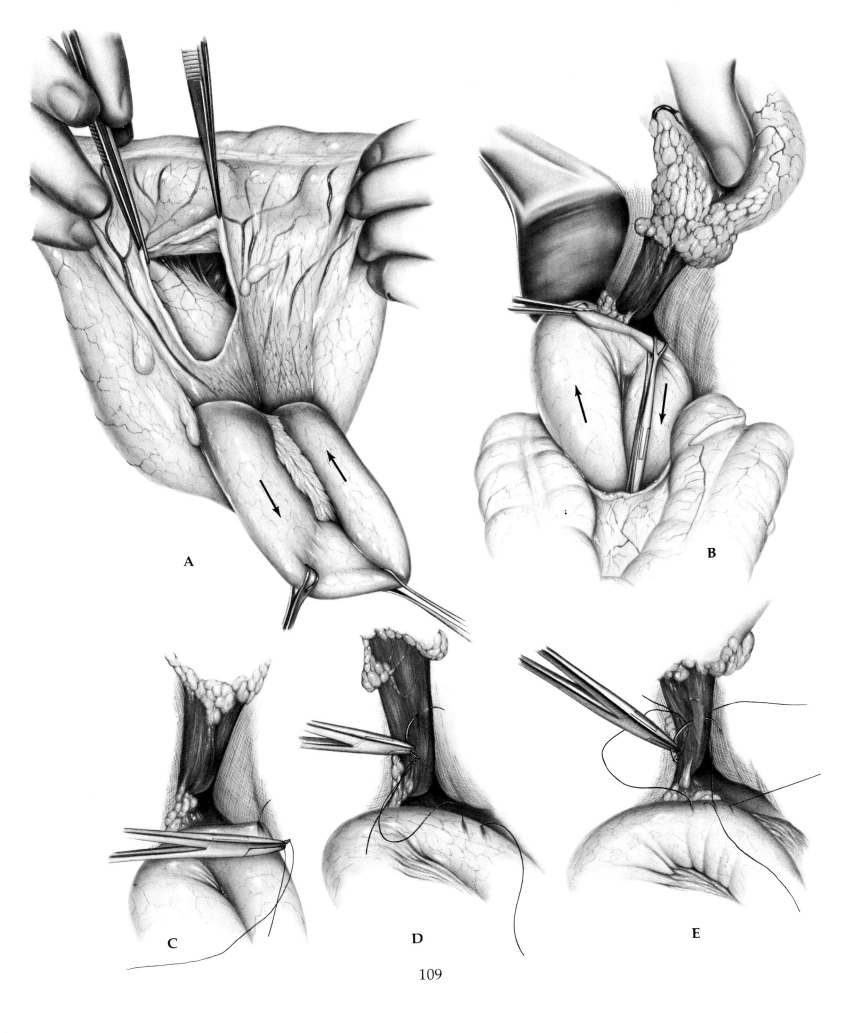

PLATE 48 • TOTAL GASTRECTOMY—cont'd

A As the suture line is continued, the horizontal placement of the sutures in the jejunum is shown.

B The esophageal portion of each stitch is carefully aligned with the jejunal portion to avoid twisting the anastomosis.

C Care must be taken to keep the jejunal suture line exactly parallel to the long axis of the bowel.

D Ample amounts of esophageal muscle must be included in these sutures.

E With each jejunal suture the needle point should be seen to blanch the bowel as it exits, indicating penetration of the seromuscular layer.

F Note the facility of suture placement gained by not ligating the sutures until all are inserted.

G As the corner is reached, the final jejunal suture is a vertical one.

H The corner esophageal suture is inserted at a slightly oblique angle to increase the security at this important point.

I All sutures are in place and ready to be tied.

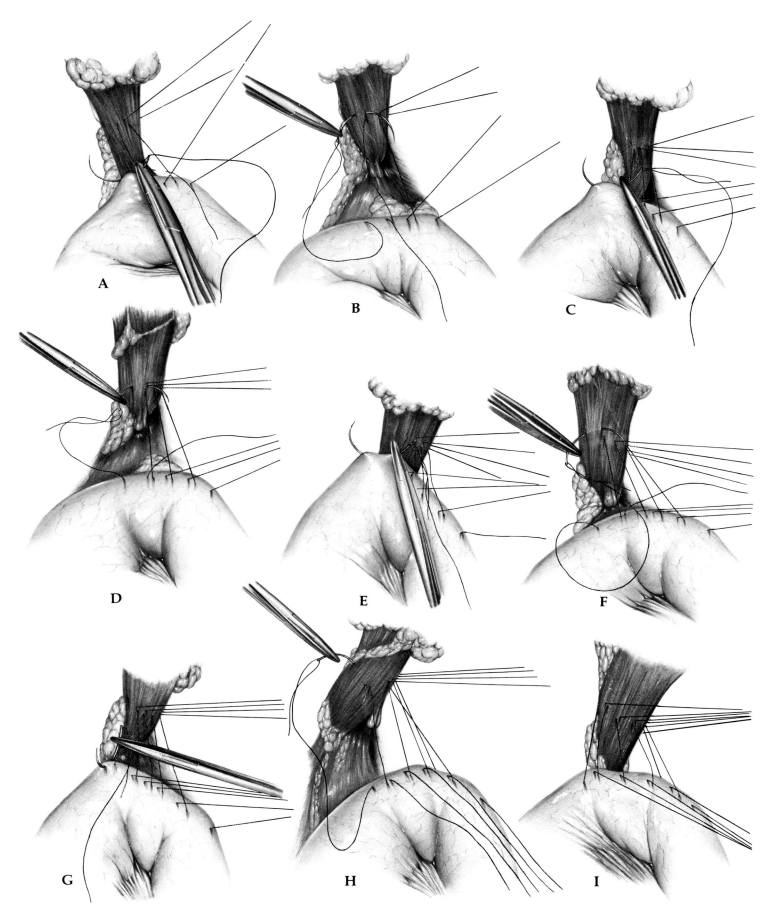

111

PLATE 49 • TOTAL GASTRECTOMY—cont'd

A The seromuscular layer at the top of the jejunal loop is incised 5 cm. along the antimesenteric border with a scalpel. Usually several small, intramural arterial bleeders need to be individually clamped and ligated prior to opening the mucosal layer. The posterior row of sutures is tied at this point.

B A fine-toothed forceps (1) elevates the mucosa, and an opening into the jejunum is made with a Metzenbaum scissors. The posterior row of sutures is now tied, approximating the posterior wall of the esophagus and jejunum.

C The opening on the jejunal side should easily admit two fingers (4 to 5 cm.).

D The posterior wall of the esophagus is incised along the posterior row of sutures and adjacent to the opening in the jejunum.

E The nasogastric tube is pulled back by the anesthesiologist until the tip is visible in the opening. After the initial opening through the posterior esophageal wall has been made with the scalpel, the opening may be extended with Metzenbaum scissors to match the opening in the jejunum. A biopsy of the open edge of the esophagus is taken when carcinoma of the stomach is the indication for total gastrectomy to ensure that tumor has not invaded the level of anastomosis.

F The corner sutures are left in place for traction. After each posterior suture is cut, an inner row of 3-0 silk interrupted sutures is placed through the seromuscular and mucosal layers of both esophagus and jejunum to complete the two layers of the anastomosis posteriorly.

G The ends of the last suture in the posterior row are cut.

H The final 3-0 silk suture is placed through all layers of both the esophagus and jejunal edges.

I The completed inner row of sutures is shown.

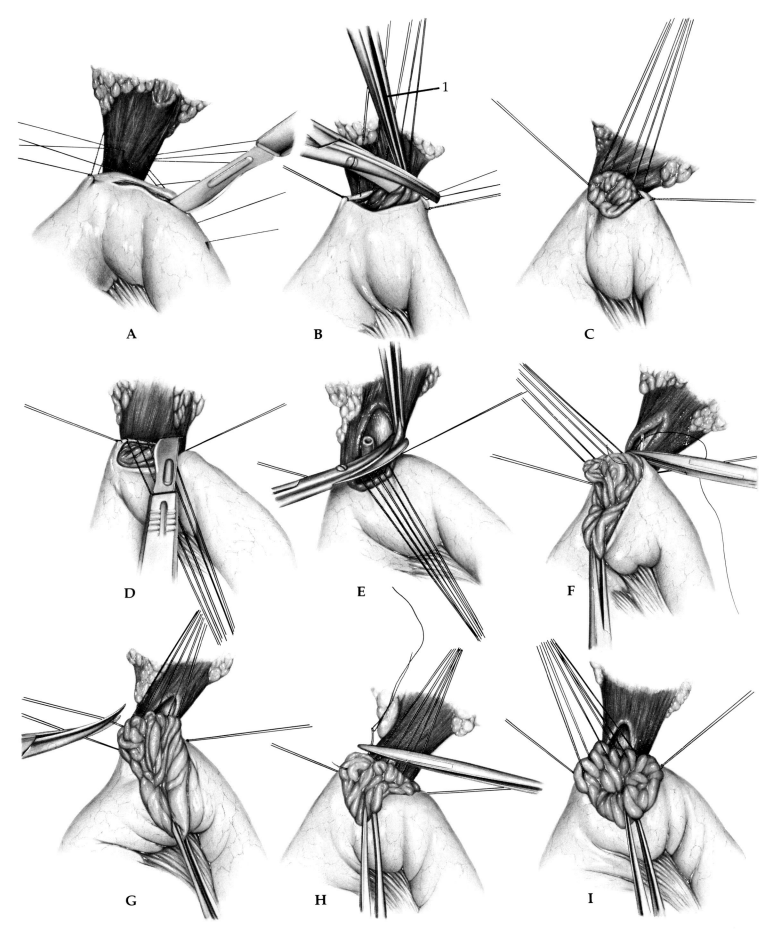

A

B

1

C

D

E

F

G

H

I

113

PLATE 50 • TOTAL GASTRECTOMY—cont'd

A The completed posterior inside row of sutures with a hemostat tagging the suture ends is shown.

B After completion of the inside row of the posterior wall of the anastomosis, the suture ends are cut. The corner sutures, marked with straight hemostats, remain for traction.

C The anterior portion of the anastomosis is started, with an inside row of interrupted sutures. The suture is placed through the jejunal side (inside out).

D The needle is then passed through the esophageal side (outside in). These sutures will be tied with the knots on the inside.

E The suture should be tied after a gentle seesaw motion and in the opposite direction of the corner traction suture. This technique will facilitate the turning in of tissue and closing the corner. The ends of each suture are cut before placing the next suture.

F The anterior inner row of sutures is continued around the corner, using the same technique.

G The suture has been passed through the opening edge of jejunum (inside out), and the needle is shown passing through the opening edge of esophagus (outside in).

H Several sutures are placed to close the opposite corner before completing the most medial aspect of the inner row. The needle is shown starting through the esophageal edge (inside out).

I The suture is then brought through jejunum (outside in), closing the far corner. Both corners should be turned early, so that the final closing sutures may be placed centrally.

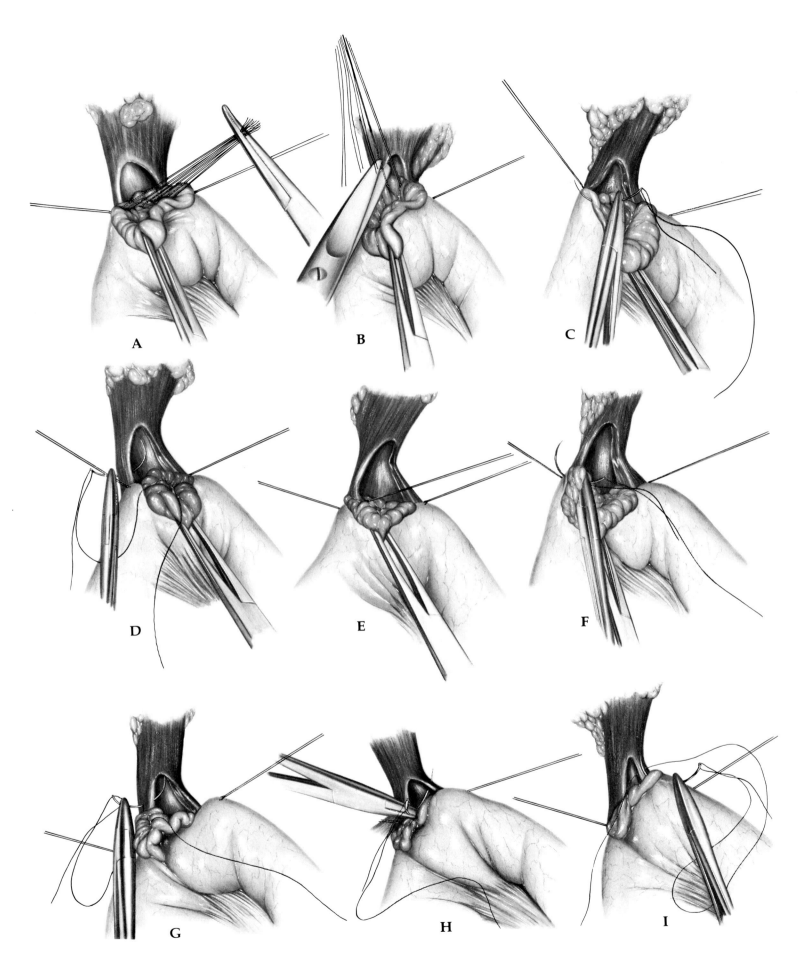

PLATE 51 • TOTAL GASTRECTOMY — cont'd

A Prior to complete closure of the opening the nasogastric tube is advanced well into the afferent limb.

B The small remnant of esophagus distal to the opening with the attached stomach is excised, and the specimen is removed.

C The closure of the anterior portion of the anastomosis is continued with interrupted 3-0 silk sutures passing through all layers. The needle is shown passing through the esophageal side (inside out).

D The suture is continued through the jejunal side (outside in). The suture is tied with the knot on the inside, and the ends are cut.

E, F The final sutures are placed, completing the inside layer of the anastomosis anteriorly.

G Anteriorly the outside row is started, using 2-0 silk interrupted mattress sutures.

H The suture bite on the esophageal side may be somewhat smaller or placed obliquely to avoid narrowing of the esophagus at the anastomosis. The more redundant jejunal wall may be folded over the inner row of sutures.

I The completed outer layer of sutures is shown. The corner traction sutures are left in place while several sutures lateral to the corners of the anastomosis are placed through the jejunum and through the diaphragm lateral to the anastomosis. Additional sutures are placed through the jejunal loop and the peritoneum of the diaphragm above the esophagus. These sutures fix the top of the jejunal loop to the diaphragm and avoid tension on the anastomosis when the patient is in an upright position.

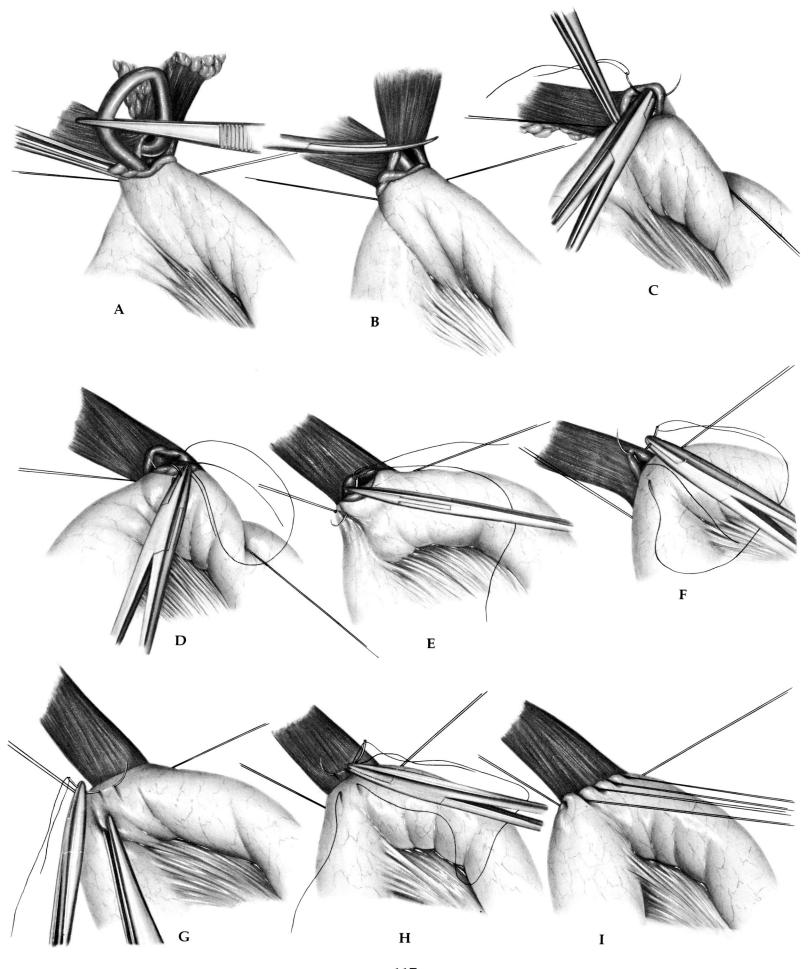

PLATE 52 • TOTAL GASTRECTOMY—cont'd

A Six centimeters distal to the esophagojejunal anastomosis, the afferent and efferent loops of jejunum are approximated by using two stay sutures 12 to 16 cm. apart. A row of interrupted 2-0 sutures is placed 1 cm. inside the antimesenteric border through the seromuscular layers of both afferent *(1)* and efferent *(2)* loops.

B A completed row of 2-0 silk interrupted sutures marks the extent of the anastomosis for a long enteroenterostomy. After placement of this row of sutures the contents of these loops are manually milked away from the area of the anastomosis. A non-gloved Scudder clamp is then placed across the mesentery and both ends of these loops. The clamp needs to be closed only 2 to 3 clicks. This clamp diminishes spillage of bowel contents and decreases mucosal bleeding when the bowel is opened.

C The muscular layer in the afferent loop is incised lateral to the first row of sutures. Any intramural arterial bleeders are ligated at this point. The muscular layer in the efferent loop is incised in a similar manner.

D The mucosal layers of both the afferent and efferent loops of jejunum are then opened with scissors. These openings extend 1 to 2 cm. short of the most proximal and distal seromuscular sutures that constitute the corner traction sutures.

E The inside row is started with through-and-through 3-0 silk interrupted sutures.

F After the first suture of the inside row has been placed, the ends of the adjacent outer seromuscular suture are cut, and the next inside suture is placed.

G After both layers of the anastomosis are completed posteriorly, the anterior inside portion is started at the far corner. The needle is shown passing through the edge of jejunum (inside out) on the efferent side.

H The suture is then continued, passing through the edge of the jejunal opening (outside in) on the afferent side. The knot is tied on the inside.

I The closure anteriorly is continued, using the inside-out, outside-in technique. A gentle seesaw motion of the suture held 180° in the opposite direction of the corner suture helps to close the corner and turn in the mucosa.

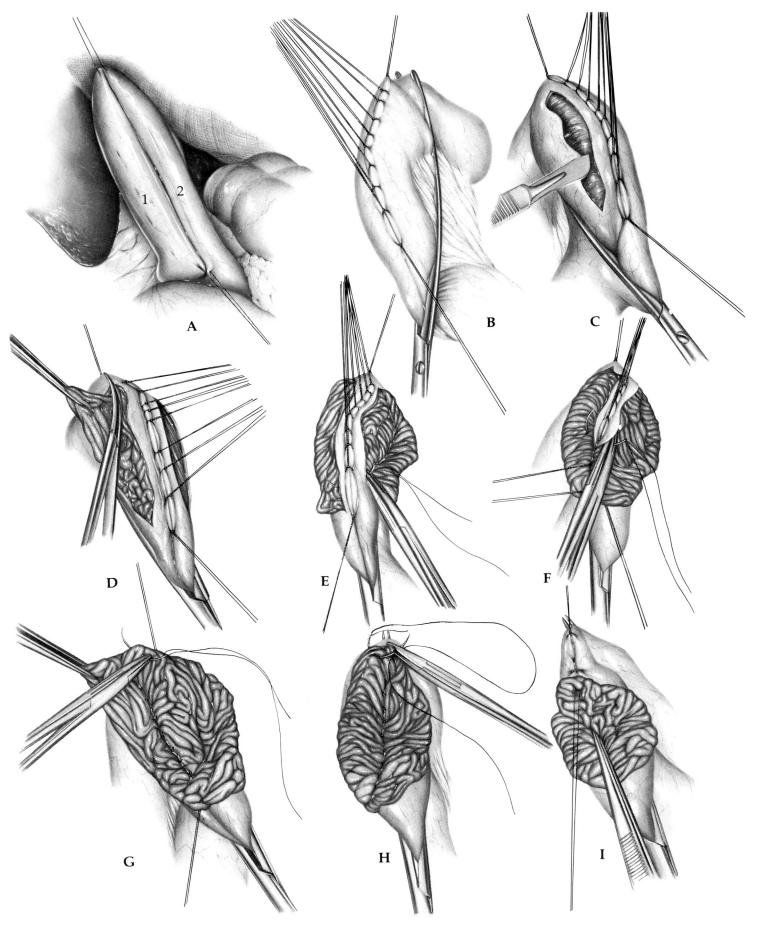

PLATE 53 • TOTAL GASTRECTOMY—cont'd

A The closure of the enteroenterostomy is continued anteriorly; the needle is shown passing through all layers of one edge of the jejunal opening (inside out).

B The suture is then passed through (outside in) the edge on the opposite side. The knot will be tied on the inside.

C The assistant holds the opposite corner traction suture 180° away from the ends of the suture the surgeon will tie.

D A gentle seesaw motion helps to turn in the mucosa before the suture is tied.

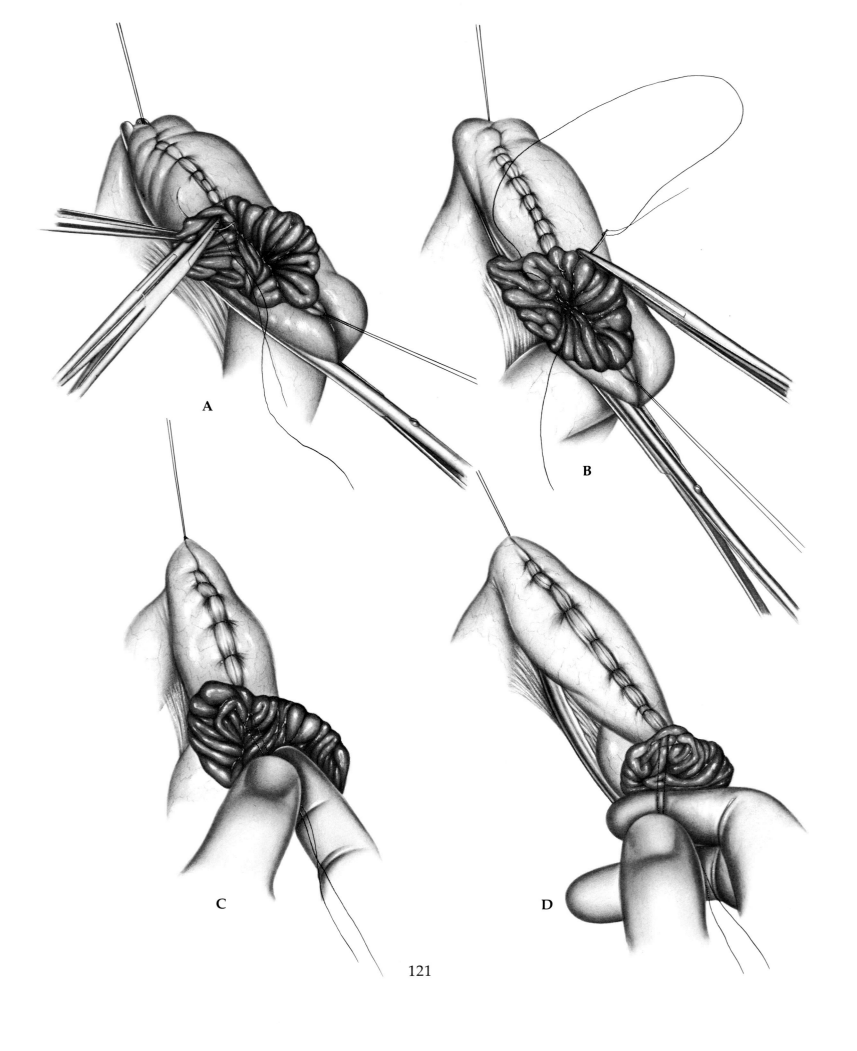

A

B

C

D

PLATE 54 • TOTAL GASTRECTOMY — cont'd

A An outer layer of 2-0 silk interrupted Lembert sutures completes the two-layer closure of the enteroenterostomy.

B Palpation ensures patency of the enterostomy. The jejunojejunostomy allows bile and pancreatic juice to pass from the proximal afferent limb into the efferent limb without passing upward and continually bathing the anastomosis in alkaline juices.

C Several 3-0 silk sutures are placed through the edge of the opening in the transverse mesocolon and the walls of jejunal loop.

D The completed closure of the opening in the mesocolon is shown. Closure of the opening by fixing the jejunal limbs to the mesocolon avoids an obvious source for an internal hernia and prevents twisting of the jejunal loop.

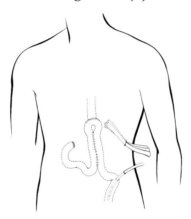

At the conclusion of the esophagojejunal anastomosis and complementing jejunojejunostomy, a distal feeding jejunostomy is constructed (Plates 55 to 57). This allows for an early feeding program. Three Penrose drains are routinely placed within 4 to 5 cm. of the esophagojejunal anastomosis. These drains are brought out through a stab wound in the left lateral flank. An osterized diet, dilute at first, may be started through the feeding jejunostomy when peristalsis returns. An oral diet is usually not started for 1 to 2 weeks. Prior to starting the oral diet, an esophagram is done to check for any leaks at the anastomosis. A leak at the esophagojejunal anastomosis may occur and persist for weeks. If the anastomotic area is properly drained, the patient may be fed via the jejunostomy tube, and nutritional balance may be maintained. One should maintain a conservative approach toward a small leak occurring at the esophagojejunal anastomosis, since the leak will close if the area is properly drained, there is no distal obstruction, and nutrition is maintained.

The surgeon bears the responsibility not only for the operation but also for the patient's postoperative nutritional maintenance. Vitamin B_{12} injections will be needed at 1- to 3-month intervals for life. An oral multivitamin preparation containing iron and calcium is prescribed. Special diets are not required, since the patient will quickly discover if between-meal snacks are necessary or if certain foods cause postprandial symptoms. Weight loss after discharge should be promptly investigated.

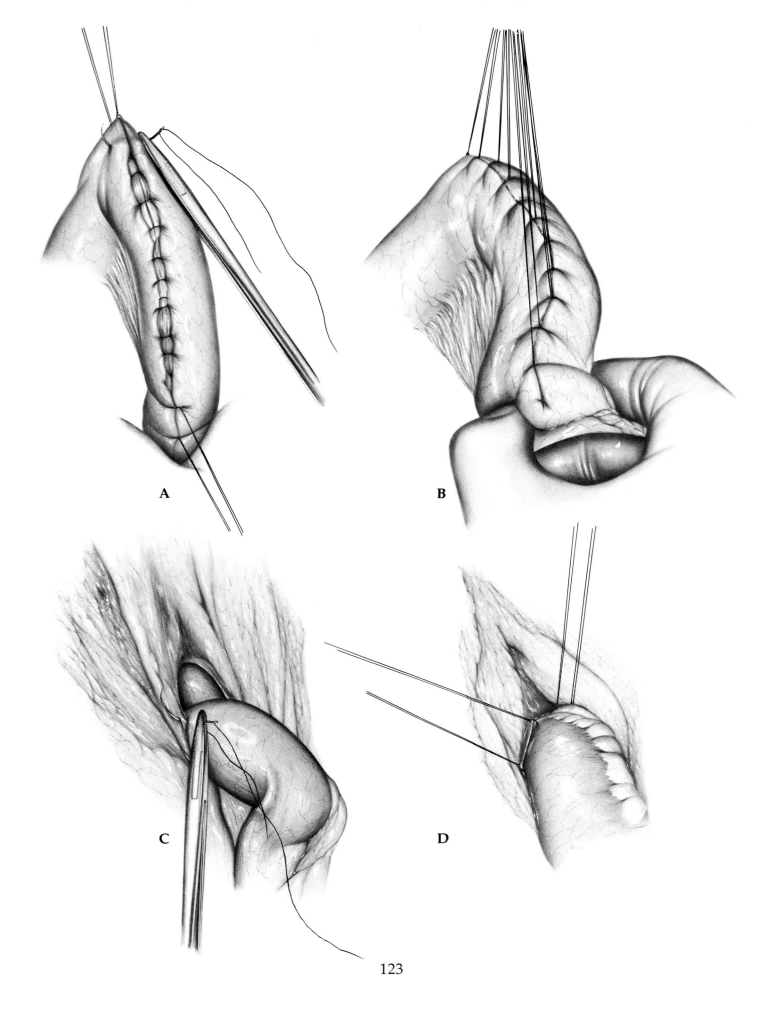

A

B

C

D

123

CHAPTER
9

Jejunostomy

Jejunostomy, an artificial communication between the proximal jejunum and the skin, is usually constructed to provide nutrition for patients unable to ingest food via the esophagus and stomach. Complicated surgical procedures involving the upper gastrointestinal tract are often an indication for jejunostomy, particularly when the jejunostomy can be utilized for early postoperative decompression and subsequent feeding if complications should arise. On rare occasions, a jejunostomy can be used to decompress a distal bowel obstruction. Even though parenteral hyperalimentation has decreased the need for jejunostomy, it remains a valuable procedure.

A Stamm type of jejunostomy (Plates 55 to 57) is recommended. The essentials of the procedure involve the placement of a soft rubber catheter into the proximal jejunum and securely anchoring the loop of the jejunum to the anterior abdominal wall. The jejunostomy must be securely fixed to the peritoneal surface to avoid leak of either intestinal contents or the feeding solution into the peritoneal cavity.

PLATE 55 • STAMM JEJUNOSTOMY

A Multiple holes are placed in a soft rubber catheter of sufficient size to prevent clogging by the feeding solution. A No. 14 French red rubber catheter is preferred.

B The holes in the catheter are cut so that they are not aligned. This technique provides maximum safety and prevents occlusion of the tube.

C A mobile loop of proximal jejunum is chosen for the jejunostomy site. It is important that this loop be completely mobile so that tension is avoided when it is secured to the anterior abdominal wall. The jejunostomy site should be at least 25 cm. distal to the liagament of Treitz. A purse-string suture is then placed into the antimesenteric border.

D A second purse-string suture is then placed approximately 0.5 cm. outside the initial suture. Note that this suture begins at about 90° from the original purse-string suture. This becomes an important technical feature when anchoring the jejunostomy. This second purse-string suture is also brought through the partial thickness of the catheter at a point at least 15 cm. from the catheter tip. This maneuver aids in preventing premature loss of the catheter from the jejunostomy site.

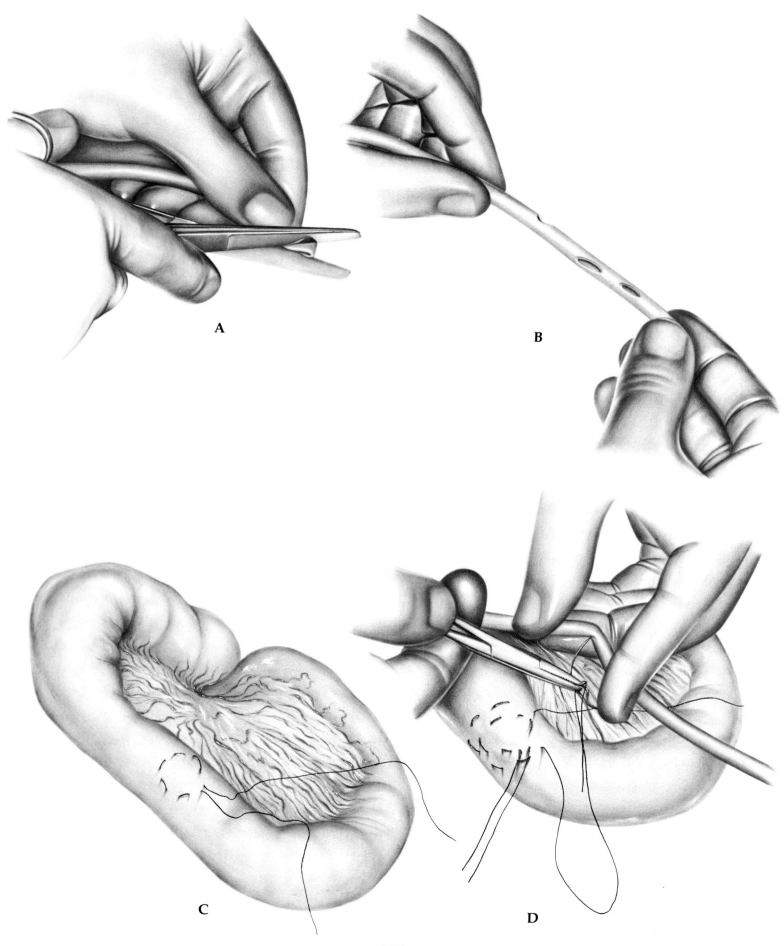

A

B

C

D

PLATE 56 • STAMM JEJUNOSTOMY — cont'd

A The double purse-string sutures are shown, and the catheter is ready for insertion into the jejunum. The suture through the tube creates no permanent problem, and after 7 to 10 days the tube can be removed or replaced easily.

B Intestinal fluid is manually expressed from the insertion site, and the assistant compresses the adjacent bowel to prevent soilage of the operative area. With suction ready, a small full-thickness incision is made into the jejunum within the innermost purse-string suture.

C The tip of the catheter is quickly inserted, and the innermost purse-string suture is tied.

D After the second purse-string suture is secured, the jejunostomy is ready for anchoring to the peritoneum.

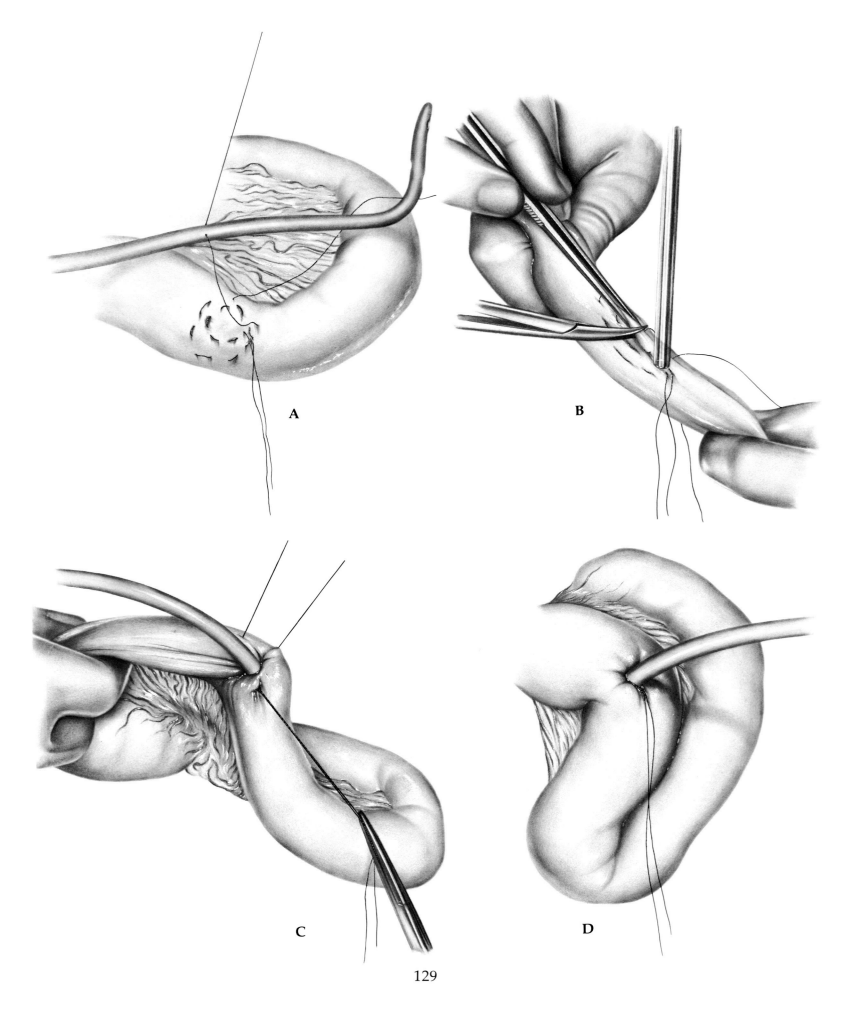

A

B

C

D

PLATE 57 • STAMM JEJUNOSTOMY — cont'd

A The fascial layers of the abdominal incision are secured with clamps and are placed on even tension. A small stab wound is made lateral to the incision.

B The end of the catheter is pulled out through this stab wound. Tension on the peritoneum and fascia allows accurate alignment of all edges of the abdominal wall.

C The jejunostomy site is then secured to the peritoneal surface, utilizing the purse-string sutures and as many separate interrupted sutures as required for secure fixation.

D The jejunostomy is completed. Some surgeons prefer to bring the jejunostomy catheter through an adjacent portion of omentum.

Feedings through the jejunostomy should not be attempted until the return of normal bowel activity. When feedings are contemplated, the catheter should be gently irrigated with saline solution. Fresh jejunostomies can seldom tolerate high-caloric feedings immediately. The initial feedings should be intermittent, low-caloric, and small in volume. Boiled skim milk, initially progressing through various dilutions of commercial high-caloric feedings, proves most satisfactory. Emulsions of high-protein, high-caloric meals can be infused with the aid of food pumps. Care must be exercised to administer supplemental fluids to avoid the consequences of infusing hyperosmolar high-protein feedings. Diarrhea can be easily controlled by varying the caloric content and by administering antidiarrheal medication with the feedings.

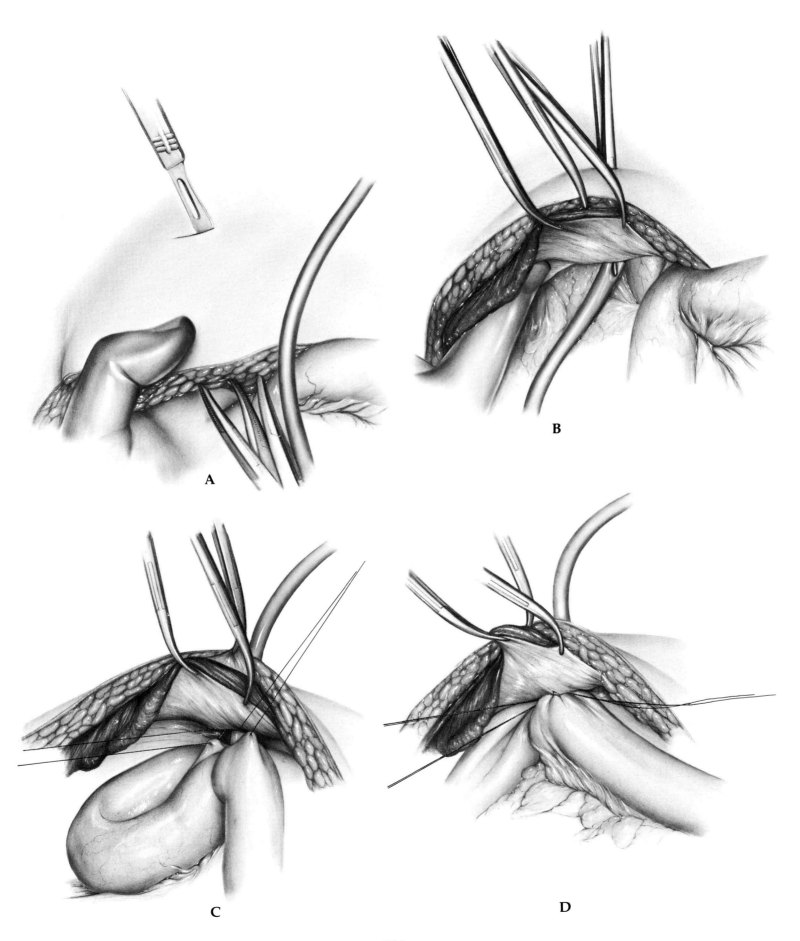

A

B

C

D

CHAPTER
10

Splenectomy for iatrogenic injury or incidental to distal pancreatectomy

The indications for an elective splenectomy have decreased during the past decade; however, the need for this procedure still arises, especially in cases of hypersplenism and in hemolytic anemia that cannot be controlled medically. The following method of ligating the splenic artery as well as the mobilization of the organ is used when removing the spleen during a total gastrectomy for carcinoma of the stomach and for traumatic rupture of the spleen. Many of the techniques of mobilization are of value in obtaining the splenic vein in preparation for splenorenal shunts.

A review of the anatomic relationships of this region will be undertaken before proceeding with the description of the operative procedure. The structures of the hilum may be considered as a single three-layered structure. The anterior layer is the gastrosplenic ligament. This structure carries the short gastric arteries that may on occasion be very short indeed. Care must be taken to avoid gastric injury and serious complications that will be discussed under the operative procedure. The posterior layer is the splenorenal ligament that is formed by the congenital fusion of two layers of peritoneum. The fused layers compose an avascular plane that can be separated by blunt dissection, although some tough fibrous bands are occasionally encountered. The middle layer would be the splenic artery and vein.

PLATE 58 • SURGICAL ANATOMY OF THE SPLEEN

A This drawing demonstrates the cross-section anatomy of the area. The anterior layer *(1)*, or the gastrosplenic ligament, is shown. The previously mentioned posterior layer *(2)*, or splenorenal ligament, is shown with the avascular plane indicated by the dark line. The splenic vessels are shown in the middle *(3)*. The tail of the pancreas *(4)* is quite near the splenic hilum.

Inset The avascular plane *(2)* is opened to allow easy access to the hilum, or middle layer, containing the splenic vein, artery *(3)*, and tail of the pancreas *(4)*. One can appreciate how easily the tail of the pancreas may be injured during splenectomy. After the anterior and posterior layers have been divided, the spleen becomes extremely mobile and can be rotated anteriorly into the operative field, making the dissection of the splenic vessels much easier and safer.

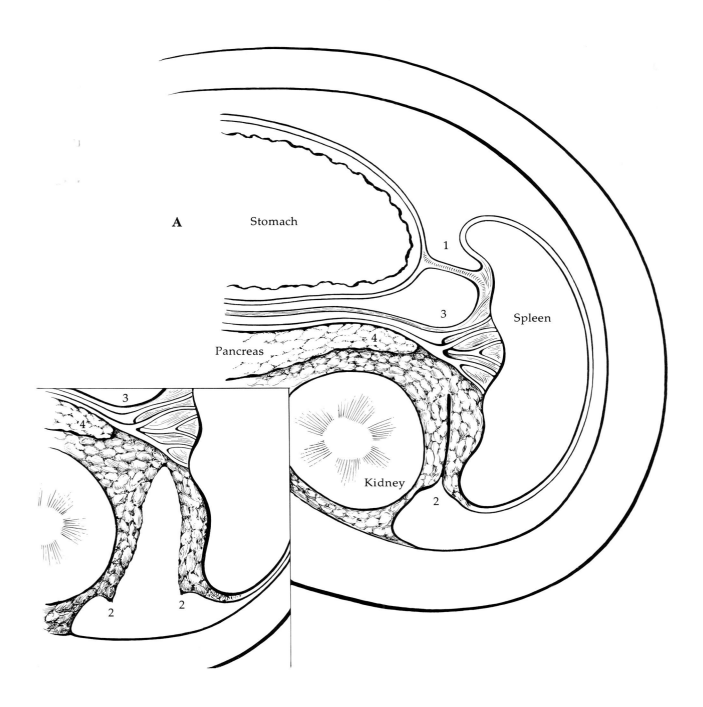

Stomach

1

3

Spleen

Pancreas

4

Kidney

2

3

4

2

2

PLATE 59 • SPLENECTOMY

The preoperative preparation is much the same as for a subtotal gastrectomy, that is, insertion of a Levin tube into the stomach prior to anesthesia and the preoperative administration of intravenous fluids. The positioning on the operating table is the same as used for all upper abdominal surgery (Plate 1, *A*); the patient is placed with the kidney rest under a line drawn through the midcostal region. By raising the kidney rest, the subdiaphragmatic structures are pushed inferiorly and anteriorly. The patient is placed toward the right of the table and rotated approximately 10° to 15° to the right. Another aid is placing the patient with the feet slightly downward, causing the viscera to fall into the pelvis out of the way of the operating surgeon.

The choice of incision is either left paramedian or a midline. Prior to making the skin incision, a scalpel is used to outline the intended incision. Usually, four cross-hatch marks are made approximately 5 to 6 cm. apart. These will act as landmarks for the exact reapproximation of the skin at the close of the procedure. A most important consideration of either incision is the extension up to the left side of the xiphoid. This simple but important maneuver greatly facilitates the exposure. A small artery is usually encountered at this point and will require a suture ligature of 3-0 silk. If a paramedian incision is used, after incising the anterior fascia, the rectus muscle is elevated from the posterior fascia by blunt and sharp dissection. Care must be taken to leave 2 to 3 cm. of posterior fascia on the medial aspect to ensure a strong closure. If a midline incision is chosen, these steps are not necessary.

A After the abdomen has been thoroughly explored, a large Richardson retractor *(1)* is placed under the left costal margin. The first assistant is then instructed to lift up gently. Care must be taken to avoid rib fracture. The emphasis on gentleness cannot be overstressed. Many patients will complain postoperatively of left costal pain when retraction has been too vigorous. The surgeon's left hand *(2)* is placed gently over the spleen to bring it forward. A laparotomy pad *(3)* is folded to a width of 3 to 4 inches and is inserted into the splenic fossa, between the spleen and the diaphragm, bringing the spleen inferiorly and anteriorly into the operative field. This is the first of many steps to mobilize the spleen so that when the structures in the hilum are approached, the organ will be at the anterior abdominal wall level.

B A Babcock clamp *(1)* is placed on the greater curvature of the stomach and pulled inferiorly and medially by the first assistant. A second Babcock clamp *(2)* is placed on the omentum, exerting tension on the gastrosplenic ligament. This facilitates the dissection of the "bare," or avascular area. This "bare" area is picked up with two fine tissue forceps and incised with dissecting scissors beginning inferiorly.

C The opening into the lesser sac is extended. As the vasa brevia are encountered, they are clamped between hemostats and divided. Careless application of these clamps may result in gastric injury and occasionally fistula formation. Note the proximity of one clamp *(1)* to the gastric wall.

D The gastric side of the vessel is then ligated with a 3-0 suture ligature. This step is extremely important. A simple ligature may slip off postoperatively, if the stomach becomes distended, and may lead to severe hemorrhage requiring an emergency operation.

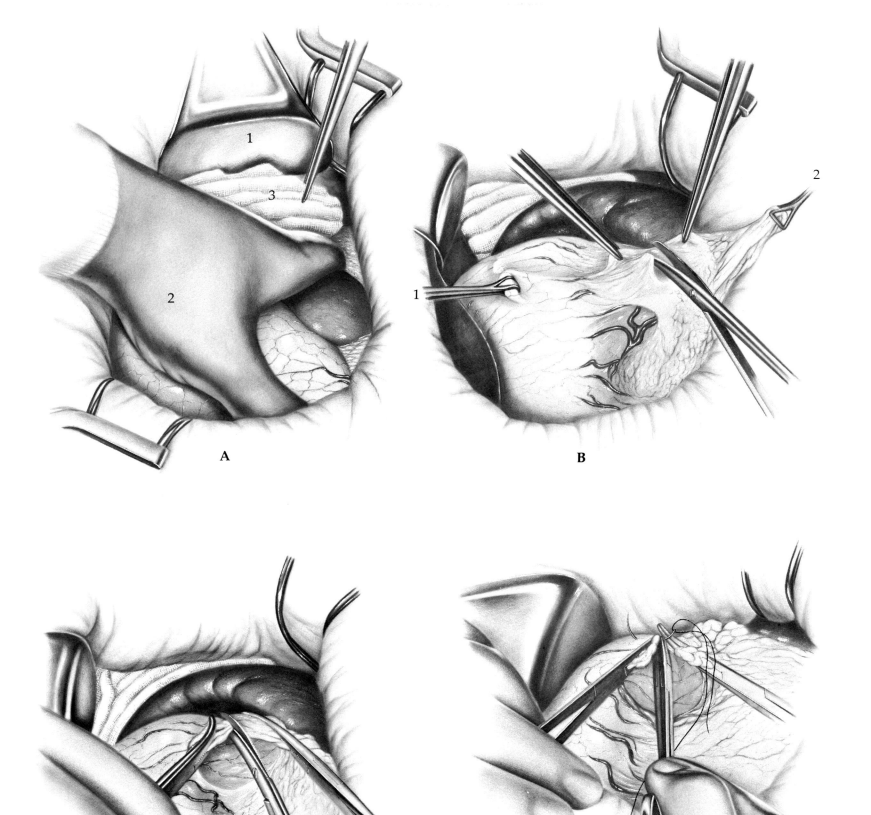

PLATE 60 • SPLENECTOMY — cont'd

A The gastrosplenic ligament division is continued, working from the inferior medial aspect of the spleen toward the superior medial aspect and dividing the tissue between the spleen and the stomach.

B Again the application of hemostats on the gastrosplenic ligament is demonstrated, pointing out the proximity of a hemostat *(1)* to the greater curvature of the stomach *(2)*.

C At this point the entire gastrosplenic ligament has been divided, exposing the pancreas *(1)* in the lesser sac. By palpating along the superior margin of the pancreas, the splenic artery is encountered. With a right-angle clamp the splenic artery is dissected from the superior aspect of the pancreas, and a suture is shown being inserted in the jaws of the clamp.

D The suture is withdrawn underneath the splenic artery, and the artery is ligated. This aspect of the procedure is dealing with hemolytic anemia now allows for the beginning of transfusion without the risk of precipitating hemolytic crisis. It also lessens hemorrhage during the remainder of the procedure.

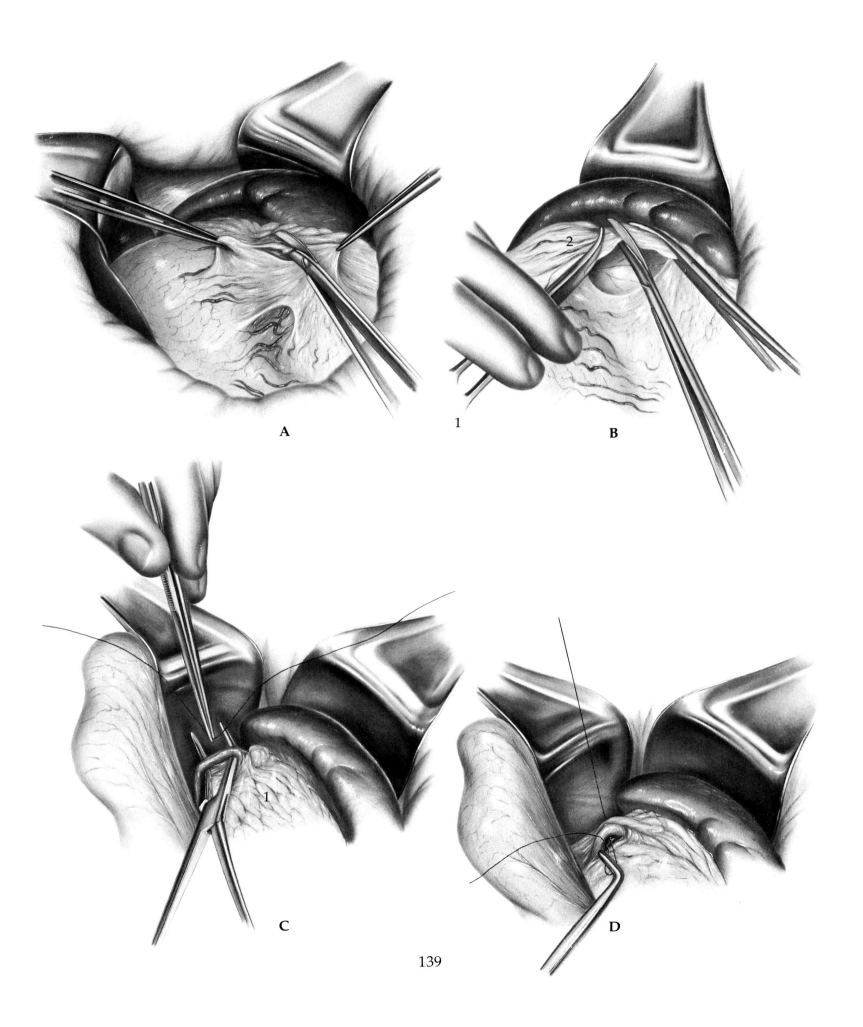

PLATE 61 • SPLENECTOMY — cont'd

A After the division of the gastrosplenic ligament has been completed and the splenic artery has been ligated, the laparotomy pad previously inserted superior and posterior to the spleen is removed. The spleen is then rotated medially and inferiorly, exposing the splenorenal ligament. This is usually an avascular plane and can be carefully divided with the scissors.

B After the incision in the posterior layer of the splenorenal ligament has been completed, finger dissection is then used to expose the splenic vessels (1) as they enter the hilum of the spleen from the posterior aspect.

C After the posterior mobilization of the spleen has been completed, the organ may now be delivered into the abdominal incision. Note the wrinkled appearance of the organ that results from having ligated the splenic artery. The arterial ligation makes the organ less tense and more safely manipulated.

D The spleen is now rotated so that the anterior aspect of the hilum is visible. The remainder of the gastrosplenic ligament is now seen (1).

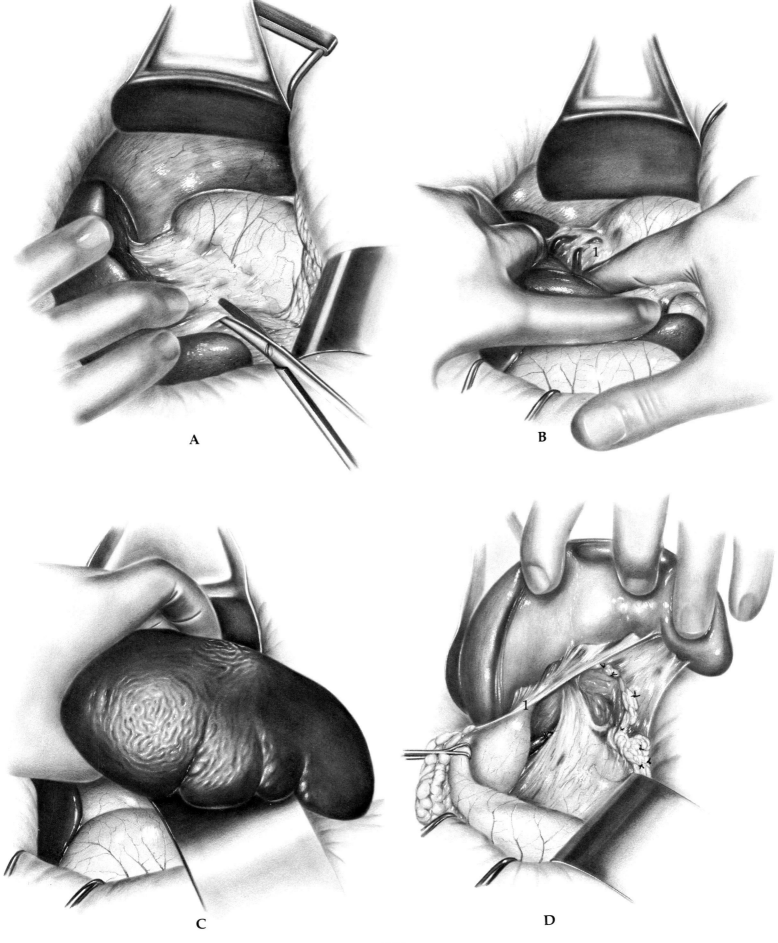

PLATE 62 • SPLENECTOMY—cont'd

A The division of the remaining portion of the gastrosplenic ligament is now completed.

B The short gastric vessels are suture ligated, with the sutures placed through the superficial layers of the gastric wall.

C Suture ligatures are preferred on the splenic side of the short gastric vessels to avoid bothersome intraoperative hemorrhage.

D The final attachment of the spleen to the stomach is divided. This step is facilitated by the use of right-angle clamps.

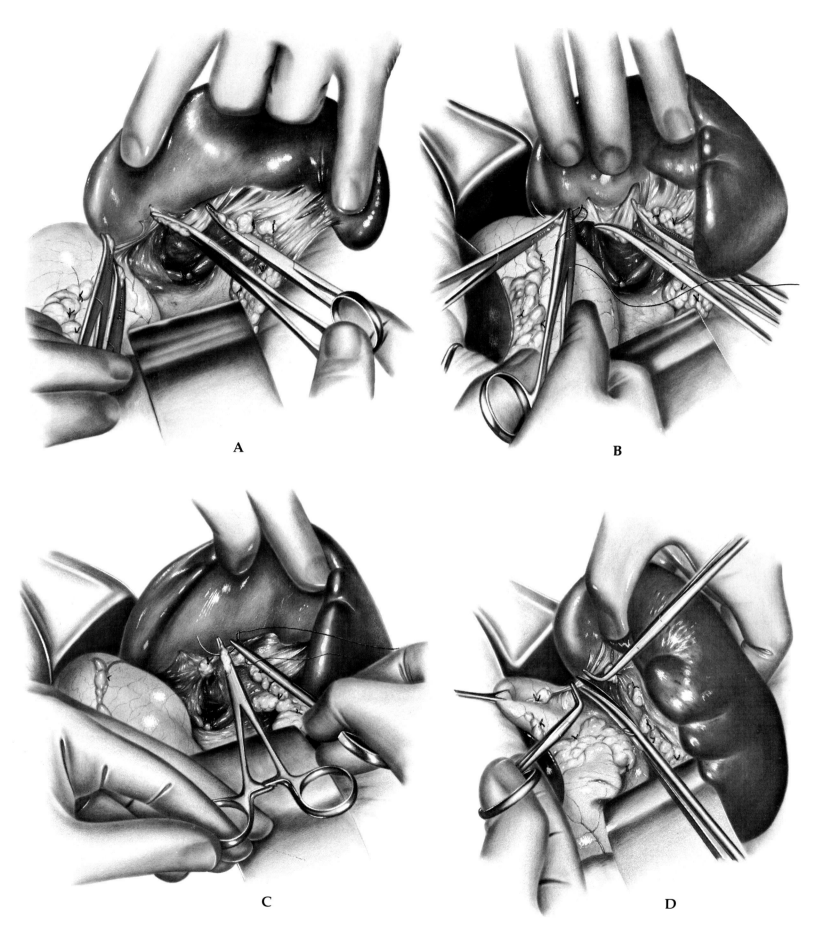

A

B

C

D

PLATE 63 • SPLENECTOMY — cont'd

A After the spleen has been completely freed from the stomach, the remainder of the splenic hilum is divided between hemostats. Note that the pancreas *(1)* is elevated with the hilar tissue.

B Suture ligature is recommended for the hilar tissue, and care must be taken to avoid pancreatic injury.

C With a curved hemostat *(1)* the previously ligated splenic artery is dissected.

D After the artery has been carefully isolated, it is doubly clamped. Branches from the pancreas to the distal splenic artery result in bothersome bleeding if the vessel is not doubly clamped.

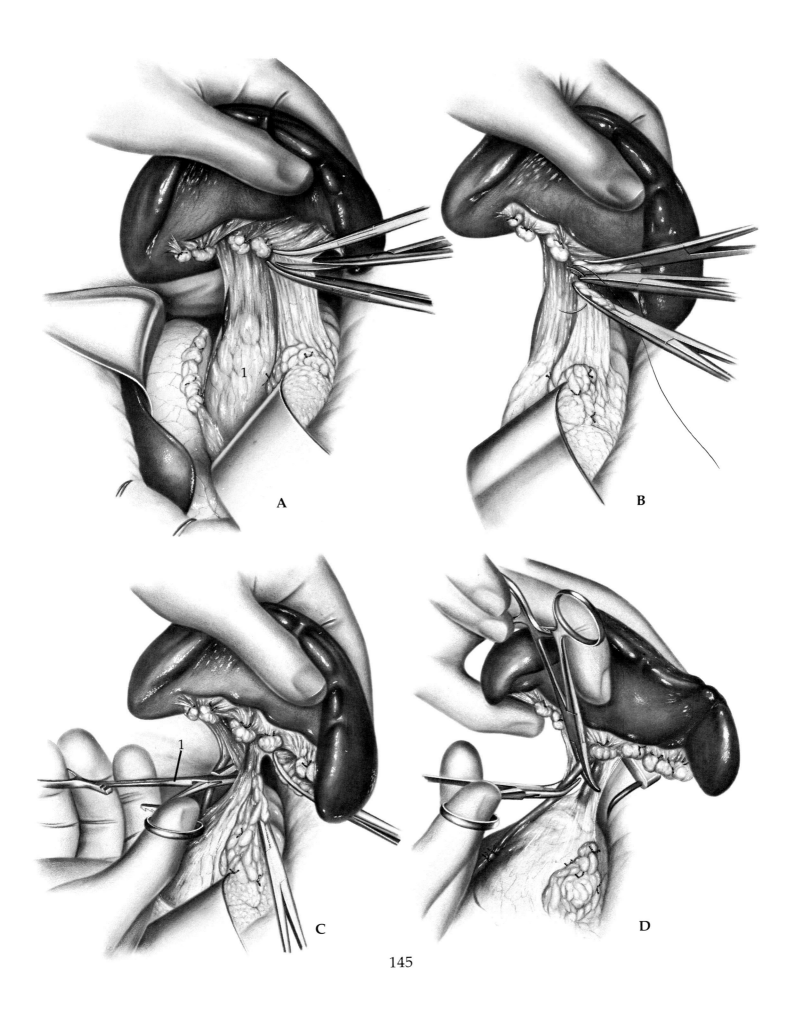

A

B

C

D

145

PLATE 64 • SPLENECTOMY — cont'd

A The splenic artery having been divided, three clamps are placed on the splenic vein, and the vessel is divided. The spleen may now be removed.

B The final step involves a free tie followed by distal suture ligature. The splenic fossa is inspected, and any small bleeding points are suture ligated. Drainage is not required.

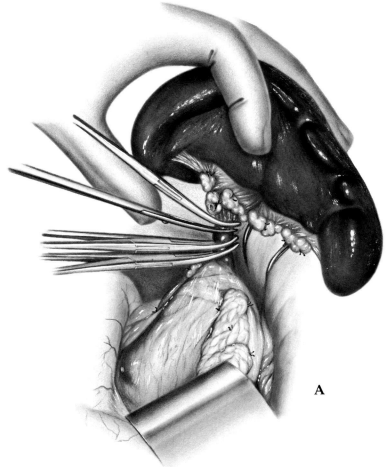

A

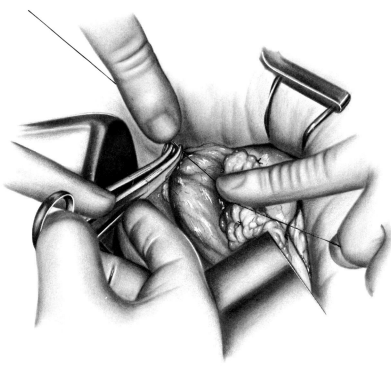

B

147

CHAPTER

11

Lymph node biopsy

Mesenteric lymph node biopsy is an extremely useful but potentially hazardous diagnostic procedure. The hazard lies in the risk of hemorrhage into the areolar tissue of the leaves of the mesentery. Once hemorrhage has occurred, search for the bleeding vessel may result in injury to mesenteric vasculature and intestinal infarction. The method described eliminates the hazard.

PLATE 65 • MESENTERIC LYMPH NODE BIOPSY

A A gauze sponge (1) is used to immobilize the node to be removed. With the sponge in the surgeon's left hand, the node to be removed is elevated with moderate tension. A scalpel is used to carefully incise the peritoneum over the node.

B After the overlying peritoneum has been excised, a curved clamp is closed about the base of the node. The node is extruded above the clamp.

C A small amount of tissue adjacent to the node is grasped with the forceps, and the scalpel is used to excise the node. This technique avoids distortion of the nodal architecture.

D The node having been removed and placed in fixative, a suture ligature of 3-0 silk is placed beneath the hemostat.

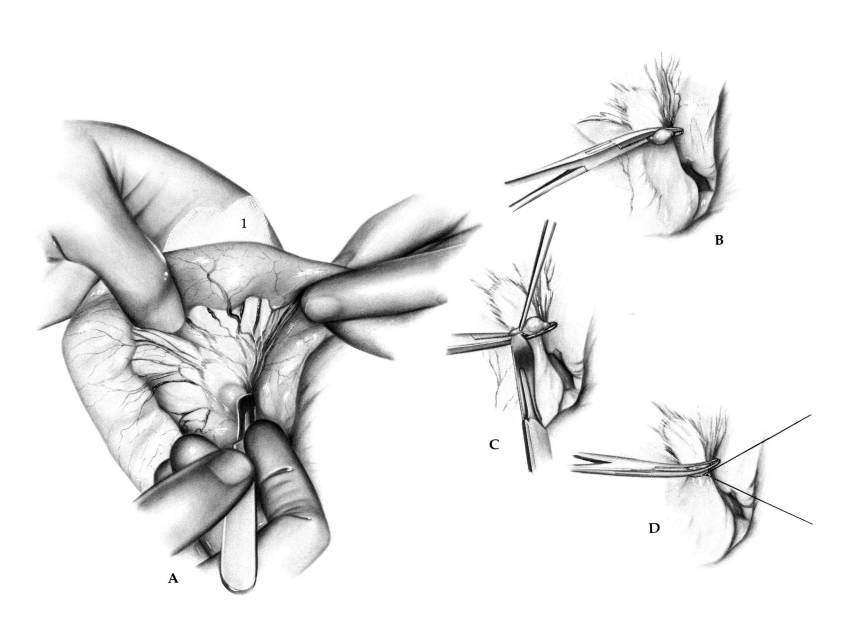

12

Distal pancreatectomy

Aside from the periampullary tumors afflicting the pancreas and adjacent organs, islet cell tumors of the pancreas may be quite difficult to find. The tumors are often small and buried in the depths of the organ, and their consistancy is not strikingly different from that of the surrounding pancreatic tissue, which makes palpation of small tumors often difficult. The following surgical procedure describes the method for thoroughly exploring the pancreas in the search for such a small tumor and for resection of the distal pancreas.

PLATE 66 • RESECTION OF TAIL OF PANCREAS

A Previous dissection has resulted in opening of the lesser sac in the method described for hemigastrectomy (Plates 6 to 8). After the stomach has been reflected superiorly *(1)* and the colon inferiorly *(2)*, exposure of the pancreas *(3)* in the lesser sac is quite easy. The dissection of the pancreas is begun by making an incision with the scissors on the inferior border of the pancreas in what is usually an avascular plane.

B After this incision has been made, finger dissection is utilized to separate the pancreas from the underlying superior mesenteric artery and vein. It is important to stay on the anterior aspect of the superior mesenteric vein, since the branches from the pancreas enter it at its sides. With careful finger dissection the pancreas can generally be separated entirely from the superior mesenteric vein posteriorly without significant hemorrhage.

C This maneuver having been accomplished, the operation proceeds to mobilization of the head of the pancreas. A Kocher maneuver has been performed and Babcock clamps *(1)* have been placed on the lateral portion of the duodenum to reflect it to the left, exposing the posterior aspect of the head of the pancreas *(2)*. The vena cava *(3)* can be seen in the depths of the wound.

D After having adequately mobilized the duodenum and the head of the pancreas, the surgeon's hand is inserted posterior to the head of the pancreas, with the thumb on the anterior aspect, and a small tumor in this area can be readily palpated. Not only can tumors in the head of the pancreas be detected in this manner, but also the occasional tumor that lies in the wall of the duodenum is best found with this maneuver.

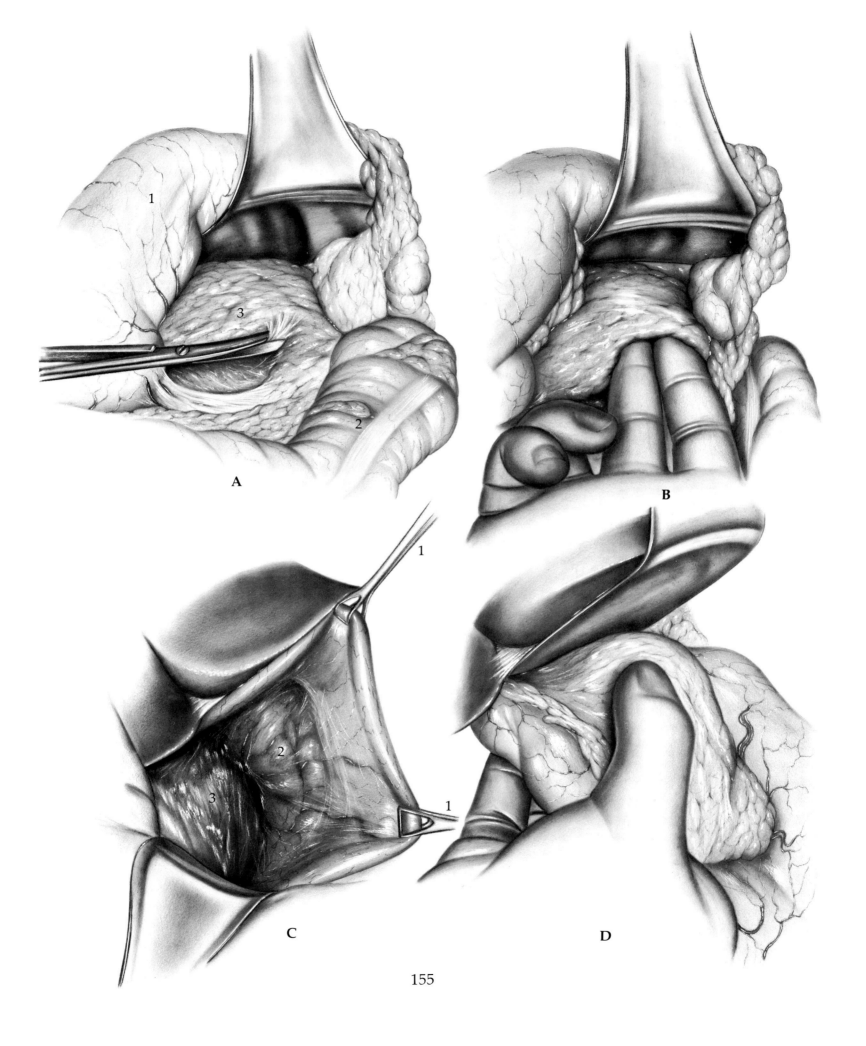

A

B

C

1

3

2

1

1

D

155

PLATE 67 • RESECTION OF TAIL OF PANCREAS—cont'd

A With the surgeon's right hand grasping the duodenum and the fingers of the right hand posterior to the head of the pancreas, the index finger is insinuated along the distal part of the lesser curvature of the stomach, and a small ulcerogenic tumor *(1)* can be seen elevated. Prior to this maneuver the tumor could not be felt. Again note the Babcock clamp that is on the area of the lesser curvature of the stomach at about the pylorus.

B The duodenum has been allowed to return to its original position, and the surgeon's middle finger is inserted from the superior aspect of the pancreas posterior to the neck of the gland as the organ is dissected free along its inferior border. Again this is frequently a plane of little vascularity, and significant hemorrhage is rarely encountered. Recall that the superior mesenteric vessels are posterior to the surgeon's middle finger.

C After the pancreas has been freed entirely inferiorly, two of the surgeon's fingers are now inserted underneath the gland, and the pancreas is elevated from its retroperitoneal position. Clamps *(1)* are placed across the tissue just distal to the tail of the pancreas. This tissue is divided and the sutures ligated. The splenic artery and vein are contained within this pedicle, and double ligature provides the safest method for management of these large vessels.

D Once the splenic vessels have been divided, the entire distal pancreas is mobile and can be elevated as seen here. A few filmy attachments of areolar tissue to the posterior aspect of the gland are divided as shown. This maneuver results in mobilization of the entire distal pancreas from the hilum of the spleen to the mesenteric blood vessels. This portion of the pancreas represents about one half the total mass of the gland and can generally be resected without metabolic consequences such as diabetes or pancreatic exocrine insufficiency.

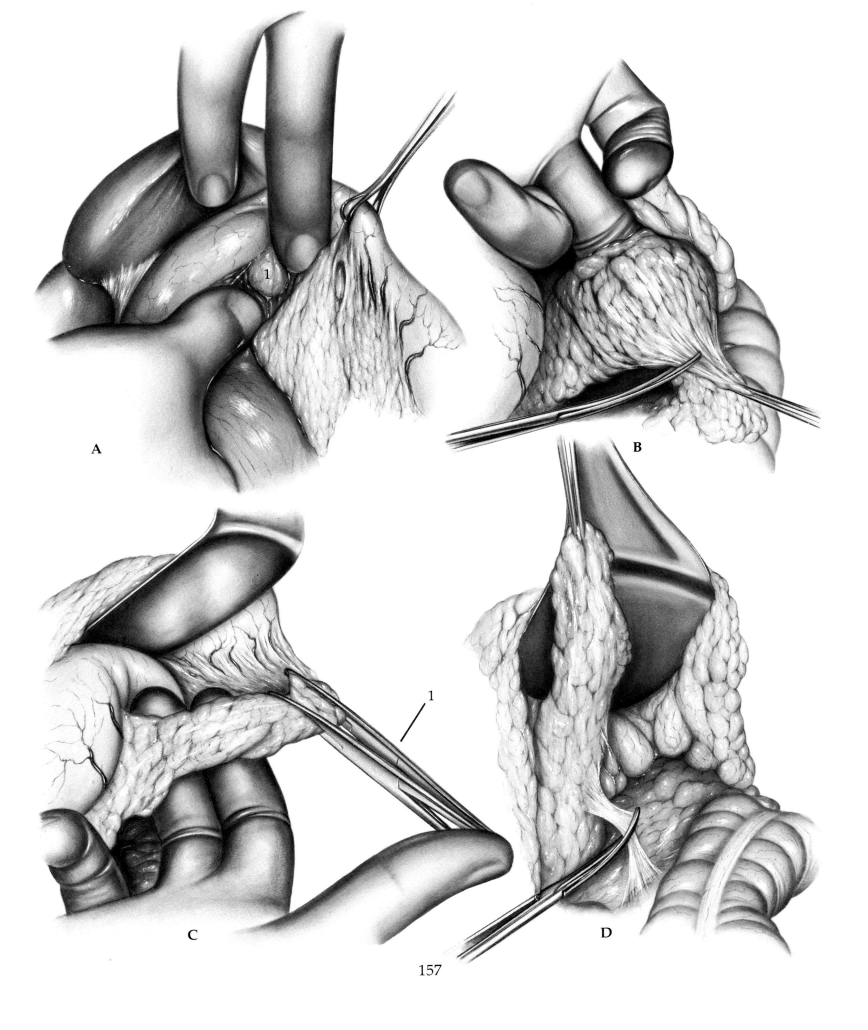

A

B

1

C

1

D

157

PLATE 68 • RESECTION OF TAIL OF PANCREAS—cont'd

If distal pancreatectomy has been elected, it is necessary to religate the splenic vein and artery in an area more proximal to that where it has previously been divided.

A The splenic artery is shown being dissected along the superior aspect of the pancreas; it is grasped between hemostats *(1)*.

B After the splenic artery has been divided, a suture ligature is used to control the proximal end of the vessel; 3-0 silk is satisfactory for this maneuver. The distal end of the transected splenic artery is then simply ligated and will be removed with the specimen. Note that the clamp *(1)* left on the tissue at the distal end of the pancreas is useful in manipulating the gland.

C After this splenic artery has been divided, the distal portion of pancreas is elevated, and a noncrushing vascular clamp *(1)* is placed across the pancreas at the site of its intended resection. The splenic vein *(2)* can be seen coursing through the midportion of the pancreas.

D The scalpel is used to transect the pancreas, and the proximal end of the gland is held within the jaws of the noncrushing clamp. The use of this kind of clamp avoids destruction of pancreatic tissue while preventing any significant hemorrhage from the transected end of the gland.

Inset After the distal portion of the pancreas has been resected, the surgeon places the specimen on a dry sponge and with the scalpel sections the organ in approximately 5 mm. slices, beginning at the site of transection and proceeding to the tail of the gland. This will allow for the detection of small otherwise undetectable pancreatic adenomas. A section of the organ is then sent to the pathologist, and a frozen section is obtained in a search for islet cell hyperplasia that is, of course, undetectable by examination of the gross specimen.

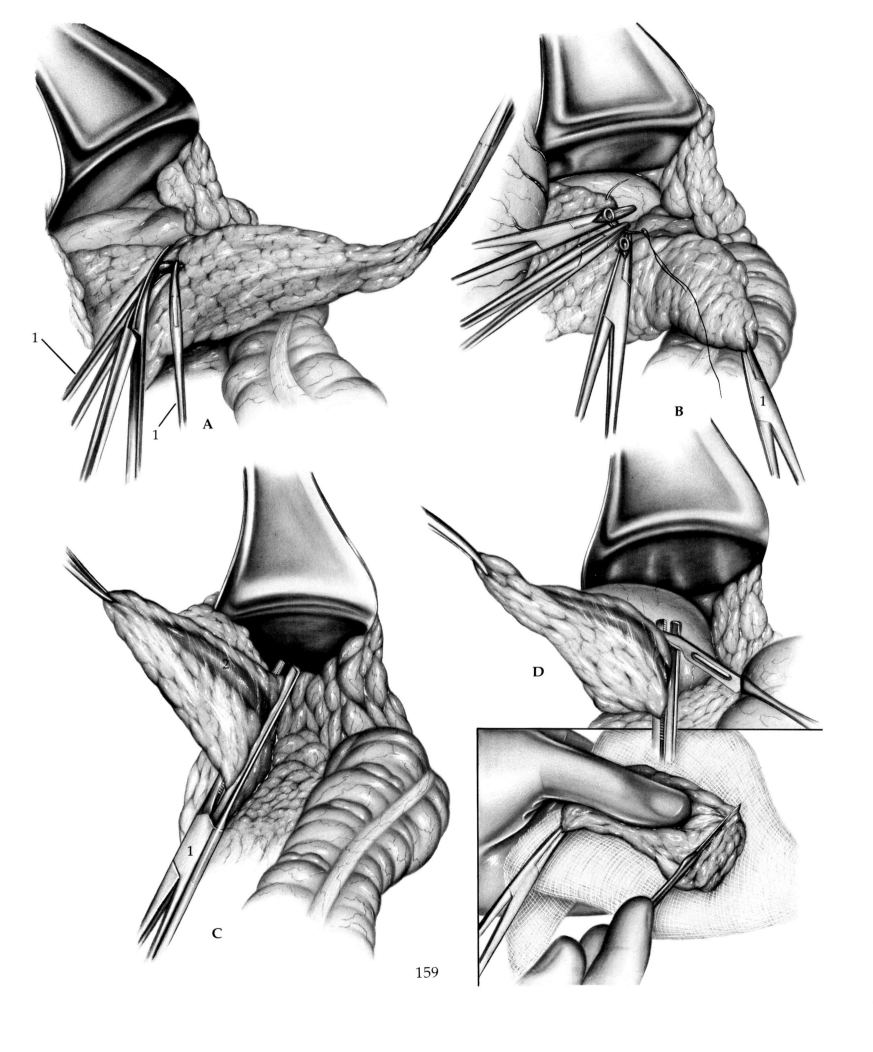

PLATE 69 • RESECTION OF TAIL OF PANCREAS—cont'd

A Traction sutures are placed *(1)* on the superior and inferior margins of the transected pancreas about 1 cm. proximal to the noncrushing vascular clamp.

B Fine French-eye needles and 3-0 silk are used to insert mattress sutures through the full thickness of the pancreas, 5 mm. proximal to the site of the clamp application. A needle is shown being inserted through the anterior aspect of the pancreas and exiting on the posterior aspect.

C The first mattress suture is being completed.

D The mattress sutures are tied as they are inserted. This suture technique is competent in controlling both hemorrhage from the cut surface of the gland and exudation of pancreatic secretions.

E The entire row of mattress sutures has been inserted and tied, and the transected end of the pancreas should now be entirely controlled. The noncrushing clamp may be removed.

F The vascular clamp has been removed, and the splenic vein that courses through the substance of the superior posterior aspect of the pancreas is now grasped with a hemostat and ligated. When this method of controlling the transected end of the pancreas is used, drainage has rarely been found to be important, and in recent years the use of a Penrose drain has been abandoned. There is no strong objection to the utilization of a drain, however. Drains made of rigid substances are to be avoided, since there is a tendancy for them to erode through the pancreatic tissue, and they are potentially more harmful than helpful.

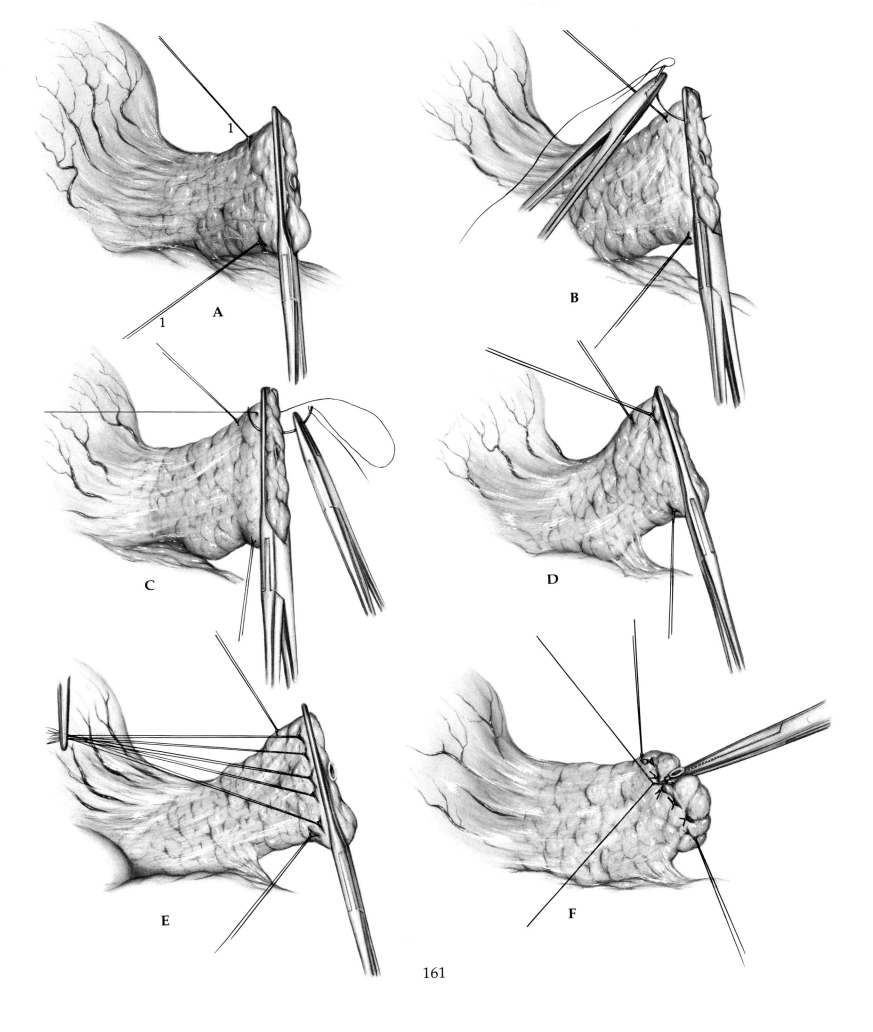

CHAPTER
13

Liver biopsy

Biopsy of the liver is a method of obtaining liver tissue for microscopic study of suspected diffuse disease of liver parenchyma or of specific lesions such as a metastatic tumor nodule. Needle biopsy is the method of choice for diffuse disease, since most pathologists prefer examining hepatic tissue obtained from the depths of the liver rather than from the leading edge. Needle biopsy samples contain less subcapsular distortion and give a truer picture of the disease process. The small samples may seem to limit needle biopsy's value; however, they adequately reflect diffuse liver disorders.

Wedge biopsy is indicated for specific hepatic lesions and in cases of suspected primary biliary cirrhosis. The method of open biopsy depicted on Plate 65 involves the preliminary placement of the hemostatic sutures and subsequent primary closure of the resultant defect.

PLATE 70 • SURGICAL BIOPSY OF THE LIVER

A The hemostatic suture should be absorbable and moderate in size (2-0 chromic catgut). A "far-near" technique is used, with the initial full-thickness suture placed approximately 3 cm. from the leading edge. The second "near" suture is placed 1 cm. from the edge.

B Care should be taken in tying this suture to prevent cutting through liver substance.

C A second hemostatic suture is placed so that the "far" stitch lies immediately adjacent to the original suture at the apex of the wedge to be removed.

D The "near" part of this second hemostatic suture is placed approximately 2 cm. from the first stitch.

E A triangular wedge of liver has been outlined by these two sutures. After the stitches are tied, a wedge of liver substance is excised with the cold knife. The specimen should be placed into a fixative immediately after gross inspection.

F The two initial sutures are tied together, approximating the liver edge. An additional stitch is being inserted for safety.

G The defect in the liver is closed on the anterior aspect of the organ.

H By using a previous suture for traction, the edge of the liver is elevated, and the posterior capsule is closed.

I If there is additional oozing from the biopsy site, hemostatic gauze is useful in stopping the bleeding. Drainage is not necessary.

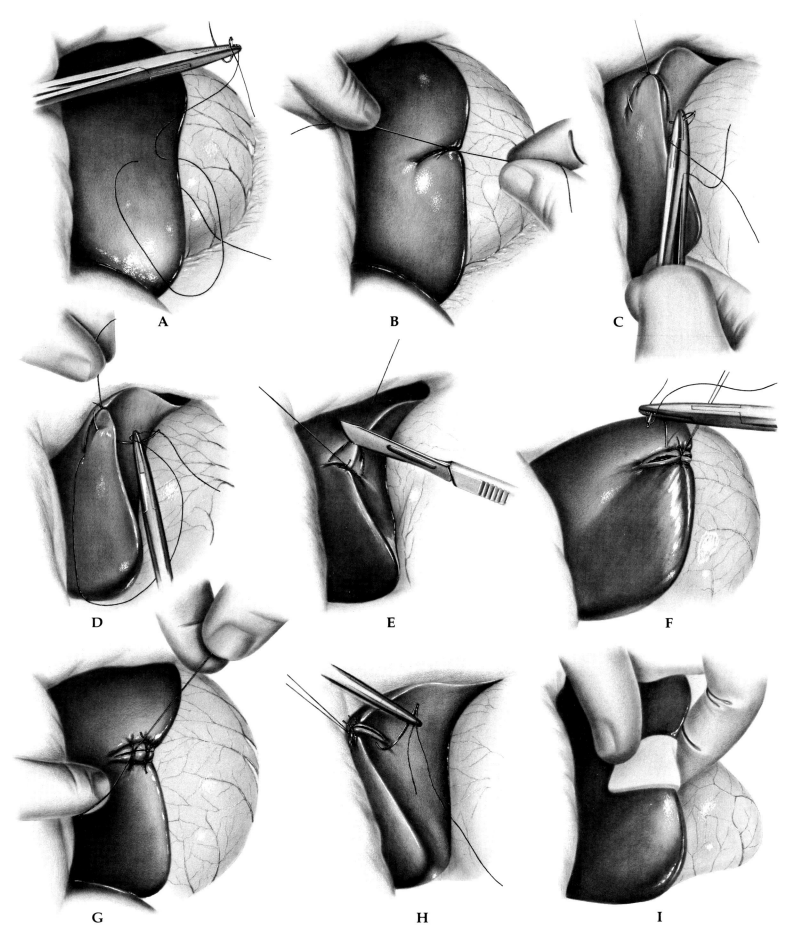